AUTHOR NOTE

All observations and opinions in this book are mine alone, written from a strictly personal perspective and not as a representative or employee of any particular ambulance service. The highest regard for patient confidentiality has been applied throughout writing this book. Patients' names, locations and other identifying features have been altered to protect privacy. In some cases, where requested, the identities of ambulance medics have also been disguised.

By the same author

Warrior Poets: Guns, Movie-making and the
Wild West of Pakistan

PARAMÉDICO

AROUND THE WORLD BY AMBULANCE

BENJAMIN GILMOUR

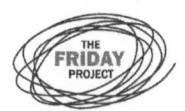

he Friday Project
An imprint of HarperCollins*Publishers*
1 London Bridge Street,
London SE1 9GF

www.thefridayproject.co.uk
www.harpercollins.co.uk

This edition published by The Friday Project 2012

First published in Australia by Pier 9, an imprint of Murdoch Books Pty Ltd in 2011

Copyright © Benjamin Gilmour 2011

Benjamin Gilmour asserts the moral right to be identified as the author of this work

A catalogue record for this book is available from the British Library

ISBN 978-0-00-749251-0

Set in Adobe Garamond Pro

*To the men, women and children working
on ambulances around the world.*

PARAMÉDICO

Benjamin Gilmour was born in Germany in 1975, but has lived most of his life in Australia where he works as an ambulance paramedic, filmmaker and writer. His first book, *Warrior Poets: Guns, Movie-making and the Wild West of Pakistan*, was published in 2008, based on his experiences directing the award-winning film *Son of a Lion*.

CONTENTS

INTRODUCTION

From the day of its invention the ambulance has attracted a magnetic curiosity from humans around the world. This vehicle racing to the scene of accidents and illness demands attention. When you hear one coming, you turn. When you watch it pass you wonder, if only for a moment, where it might be going, who is inside and what horrific mishap the patient has suffered. After fifteen years spent in the back of ambulances I've come to realise that medics and paramedics are endlessly fascinating to the public.

But despite our appeal, the truth about us is largely hidden from view. It is hidden because, in the instant we drive past we have carried our secrets away, leaving nothing more than the wail of a siren. We are hidden because the usual depiction of paramedics on film and television is mostly a fantasy. The title of hero is forced upon us, and what is lost is who we really are.

Right now, as you read this, more than a hundred thousand ambulance medics in all manner of unusual and remote locations across the planet are responding to emergencies. They are scrambling under crashed cars, carrying the sick down flights of stairs, scooping up body parts after bombings, comforting the depressed, resuscitating near-dead husbands at the feet of hysterical wives, and stemming the blood-flow of gunshot victims in seedy back alleys. A good number too are just as likely to be raising an eyebrow at some ridiculous, trivial complaint their patient has considered life-threatening. Each of these medics could fill a book just like this one, with adventures many more extreme, dangerous and shocking than those recounted here.

My fascination with the lives of people from countries and cultures other than my own is driven by my ultimate desire to understand humanity. And so I travel at every opportunity to observe how people interact, and learn why they believe what they do, how they live and how they die and how they grieve. From the age of nineteen, during periods of leave each year, I have worked or volunteered with foreign ambulance services. Whether acting as a guest or consultant, I stayed sometimes for a month, other times more than a year. Every day it has been a privilege. There are few professions like that of an ambulance worker – we have a rare licence to enter the homes of complete strangers and bear witness to their most personal moments of crisis.

Globally, the make-up of ambulance crews is varied, though it's generally agreed there are two models of pre-hospital care delivery – the Anglo-American model based on one or two paramedics per ambulance, or the Franco-German model where the job is performed by doctors and nurses. Over recent years, a number of Anglo-American systems have also introduced paramedic practitioners with skills that, until now, have been the strict domain of emergency physicians. Pre-hospital worker profiles also include drivers and untrained attendants who can still be found responding in basic transport ambulances across many developing countries. Since cases demanding advanced medical intervention represent only a small percentage of emergency calls, it would be a mistake to judge ambulance workers as 'good' or 'bad' solely on clinical ability. Consequently, I have chosen to explore the world of many ambulance workers, no matter where they are from or what their qualifications. It is true that ambulance medics are united by the unique challenges of their job. They are members of a giant family and they understand one another instantly. While the work may differ in its frequency, level of drama and cultural peculiarities, there is no doubt that medics the world over experience similar thrills and nightmares.

As a paramedic and traveller, I've enjoyed the company of my brothers and sisters in many exotic locations. I've lived with them, laughed with them and cried with them. And wherever it was I journeyed, my ambulance family not only showed me their way of life, they also unlocked for me the secret doors to their cities and the character of their people, convincing me that paramedics are the best travel guides one can hope to have.

More than a story about the sick and injured, *Paramédico* is about the places where I have worked and the people I have worked there with. It's about the men and women who have remained a mystery to the world for long enough.

So, climb aboard, buckle up, and embark with me on these grand adventures by ambulance.

OUTBACK AMBO

Australia

For two weeks I have sat here in this fibro shack along the Newell Highway listening to the ceaseless drone of air-conditioning, waiting for the sick and injured to call me. Coursework for my paramedic degree is done and all my novels are read. Now I wait, occasionally wishing, with guilt, for some drama to occur, some crisis, no matter how small, anything to break the monotony of my posting.

From time to time my mother sends me a letter or her ginger cake wrapped in brown paper. For the second time today, I drive to the post office in my ambulance.

I'm stationed in Peak Hill in central New South Wales, a town some locals might consider their whole world. But to me, a nineteen-year-old city boy with an interest in surfing and clubbing, I am cast away, marooned, washed up in the stinking hot Australian outback.

'Sorry, champ,' says the post officer. 'Nothing today.'

And so I drive my ambulance around the handful of quiet streets where nothing ever changes, where I rarely see a soul. Shutters are down, curtains drawn, doors shut. Where are they all, I wonder, these people who apparently know my every move?

I turn down towards the wheat silo and park, imagining how I would treat someone who had fallen from the top of it. After that I go to meet a flock of sheep with whom I've learnt to communicate. Much of it is non-verbal. We just stand there, the flock and I, face to face, staring quietly, contemplating what the other's life must be like. Now and then we exchange simple sounds by way of call-and-response. Whenever I think I've gone mad I remind myself that most people talk freely to their pets without a second thought.

Earlier in the year, the Ambulance Service of New South Wales sent my whole class to remote corners of the state. I understood, of course, that in our vast country with its sparsely populated interior, everyone is equally entitled to pre-hospital care. Only problem is that few applications to the service are received from people living in the bush. Instead, young, degree-qualified city recruits from the eastern seaboard end up in one-horse towns.

As I entered the Club House Hotel in Caswell Street on my first night, twelve faces textured like the Harvey Ranges turned my way, looked me up and down taking in my stovepipe jeans, my combed hair and patterned shirt. As if my appearance was not out of place enough, I foolishly ordered a middy of Victoria Bitter and the room erupted in thigh-slapping laughter. Before I ran out, a walnut of a man nearest to me leant over to offer some local advice.

'Out here, mate, it's a schooner of Tooheys New, got it?'

I never went back to the pub, at least not socially. When called there in the ambulance for drunks fallen over, I was always greeted with the same row of men in the same position at the bar, like they had never gone home. It didn't take me long to realise I'd need to find entertainment elsewhere.

In less than a month Kristy Wright, an actor playing the role of Chloe Richards on the evening soap *Home & Away,* has become the object of my affection. As the elderly will attest, a routine of the ordinary brings security of sorts, a familiar comfort, and *Home & Away* is just this for a lonely paramedic with too much time on his hands and not enough human company. Kristy is not particularly glamorous, nor is she Oscar material. Perhaps it's her likeness to my first proper girlfriend, a ballerina who ran off to Queensland, married someone else, and broke my heart. Whatever the reason, I'm deeply smitten and make sure never to miss an episode.

For a small fee I have taken accommodation in the nurses' quarters on the grounds of Peak Hill's tiny brick hospital with its single emergency bed. Adjacent to the hospital lies the ambulance station consisting of a small office, a portable shed with air-conditioning and a garage containing an F100 and a Toyota 4x4 ambulance for difficult terrain. My new home next door is a freestanding weatherboard cottage, a little rundown but quaint nonetheless. Lodging at these nurses' quarters initially sounded quite appealing to a young, single man, but the place never came with any nurses in it.

At 8 pm I ladle some lentil soup out of a giant pot I prepared earlier in the week, heating it up on the electric stove. After dinner, at 9 pm, I run the bath, making sure my blue fire-resistant jumpsuit is hanging by the door and my boots are standing to attention below, ready for the next job – if I ever live to see it, that is. Two slow weeks and I'm beginning to think they should close the ambulance station down before their assets rust away. The population plummeted a few years ago when Peak Hill's gold mine hit the water table and ceased operations. Locals left behind would disagree, but maybe ambulance stations ought to come and go with the mines.

When the call finally comes it catches me off guard, just as I knew it would, cleaving me from a deep 4 am sleep.

'Huh?' I grunt into the phone. The dispatcher in the Dubbo control room 80 kilometres away sounds just as vague.

'Okay, what we got here, let me see, ah, semi rollover on the Newell Highway six kilometres south of Peak Hill ... well, that's about all I have, mate ... good luck with it.'

I hang up, slide out of bed in my jocks, splash my face at the bathroom sink, head to the door.

Keys, keys, ambulance keys. I teeter on the remains of sleep, trying to think of where I put the keys. When I throw my legs into the jumpsuit I'm relieved to hear them jingling in a pocket. My boots are on and I'm out.

The engine of the Ford springs to life, the V8 gives a mighty roar, a call to action. Adrenalin, like petrol charging through the lines, ignites me for the fight. I flick on the red flashing roof lights, the grill lights on the front, and then, as I skid onto the highway, I let the siren rip through the stillness. There's not a car in sight, no one at all to warn of my approach, but this run is for the hell of it. I'm doing it because I can, because for two weeks I've been bored out of my brain and I'll be damned if I won't make the most of a genuine casualty call.

The Ford is a missile; eight cylinders of muscle thundering down the highway. In no time I cover the six kilometres, wishing the crash was further away for a longer drive. Last month it took me sixty minutes on the whistle travelling at speeds of 150 kilometres per hour to reach a child fallen off a horse at a remote property.

Up ahead a pair of stationary headlights in the middle of the road beam at me. They appear, at first, to be sitting higher than normal, but when I get closer I realise the semitrailer to which they belong has flipped upside down. It's a most peculiar sight.

No one has motioned me to stop. In fact, there is no one about at all, not even Doug the policeman. Further down the road I spy another truck pulled up with its hazard lights on and assume this driver must have called the job in.

The motor of the upturned semi is still idling. It's an eerie sound in the absence of any other. I decide that, for the purpose of making the scene safe and preventing an explosion, I ought to switch it off.

From what seems to have been the passenger side of the truck a steady stream of blood runs slowly to the shoulder of the road. The entire cabin of the semi is crushed and when I call out 'Hello there!' I don't even get a grunt of acknowledgement.

This is my job, I remind myself. It falls on no one else. It is precisely my duty, without further delay, to climb underneath the overturned truck, attempt to turn off the ignition and ascertain the number and condition of its occupants.

With a small torch in hand, I get down on my chest and crawl into a narrow passage about a foot high with twisted metal and shattered glass all around, my head is turned on the side, oil and bitumen brush my cheek until I reach an opening in front of me. Here I'm able to lift my head up and take a look around. When I do this my heart jumps like a stung animal as I find myself face-to-face with the driver, his head pummelled into a mushy, shapeless mess, his mouth gaping wide and a single avulsed eye glaring at me. For the first time ever I am simply too startled to shriek or utter any sound whatsoever. Confined like this makes a rapid retreat difficult. Instead, I am frozen in horror, just as the driver's face may have been in the moment before it was destroyed by his dashboard.

After a few seconds, when I regain a little composure, I reach up to the keys dangling in the ignition and turn off the engine. At the same time I see a photo of a woman and child, smiling at the camera, some birthday party. Perhaps it was the last image the man saw before exhaling his final breath.

Almost as slowly as I entered the cabin I extract myself and return to the ambulance, shaking ever so slightly, to give Dubbo control a report from the scene.

It takes Peak Hill's SES Rescue Squad five hours to remove the driver's body. Most of this is spent waiting for a crane to arrive from Parkes. I stand in the shadows clutching a white folded body bag, reluctant to join the rescue volunteers, all ex-miners and rough farmhands cursing and spitting and slapping each other on the back.

At the hospital, the nurse on duty has called in Peak Hill's only doctor, a short Indian fellow, to sign the certificate. When I unzip the body bag and pull it back, all colour drains from the doctor's face, his eyes roll into his head and he grips the wall to stop himself from passing out.

'Doc may need to lie down for a while,' I say to the nurse as she leaps forward to prevent him falling.

By the time I finish at the morgue the sun is high over the Harveys and I reverse the ambulance into the station, putting it to bed for another two weeks.

Most of Peak Hill's indigenous population lives in what is still known as 'the mission', a handful of streets on the south side of town once run by missionaries. In comparison to many Aboriginal missions in the Australian outback, the houses are fairly tidy and the occupants give us little trouble. Except for Eddy and his extended family, that is. When things become too monotonous in Peak Hill one can always rely on Eddy to get pissed, flog his missus or end up unconscious in someone's front yard. Empty port flagons line the hallway of his house, a house without a door and with every window smashed in. Half the floorboards have been torn up for firewood in the winter.

Jobs often come in spurts and on the day after the semi rollover I scoop Eddy onto the stretcher and cart him to the hospital for his weekly sobering-up. In straightforward cases like this I work alone, making sure to angle the rear-vision mirror onto the patient for visual observation. Occasionally, to be certain the victim doesn't pass away unnoticed, I attach a cardiac monitor for its regular audible blipping. This way I can keep my eyes on the road ahead.

Longer journeys are a little trickier. For these I must evaluate a patient's blood pressure every ten minutes or so by pulling over and climbing into the back. It is hardly ideal, but sometimes necessary when I'm unable to find a suitable or sober candidate to drive the ambulance for me. A strategy the service conceived many years ago was to recruit volunteer drivers from the community, people familiar with the names and location of distant cattle stations and remote dirt tracks.

Charlie, a hulk of a man with handlebar moustache and hearty belly laugh is the best on offer. Unfortunately his job as a long-haul coach driver means he's rarely in town when I need him. Perhaps one day he will join the service full-time.

As for Lionel, Peak Hill's only other volunteer officer, he is simply too crass to take anywhere at all. Unshaven, slouchy and barely able to complete the shortest string of words without adding expletives, Lionel is my last resort. Nonetheless, his job as the hospital caretaker means he torments me with racist, redneck tales and invitations to bi-monthly Ku Klux Klan gatherings held at secret locations in the Harvey Ranges. His open dislike of 'boongs' – a derogatory term for Aboriginal people – is another reason I don't take him on jobs in the mission. Lionel's most beloved pastime is 'road kill popping', which involves intentionally driving over bloated animals with his Ford Falcon in order to hear them 'pop' under the chassis. Worse still, less than a month after my arrival in Peak Hill, he snatched a snow-white cooing dove from the eaves of the ambulance station and ripped its head off, whining about the 'pests' inhabiting the hospital rafters. This callous act prompted me to slam the door in his face.

When my family drives up from Sydney to pay me a visit I take them to the Bogan River, just out of town. It's a sorry little waterway but there are several picnic spots to choose from. In the shade of a snow gum we spread out a tartan blanket. My mum unwraps her tuna sandwiches and pours out the apple juice while my dad reflects on the subjects of solitude, meditation, Jesus in the desert. My sister and brothers are not normally so quiet and I sense everyone feels a bit sorry for me, as if I have some kind of incurable disease, all because I'm stuck here in Peak Hill.

Later that night, as no volunteer drivers are available, my dad offers to join me on a call to the main street. He's still tying the laces of his Dunlop Volleys in the front seat when I pull up at the address. Above the newsagent, in a room devoid of any furniture, an eighteen-year-old male is hyperventilating and gripping his chest. The teenager is morbidly obese for his age, thanks to antidepressants and a diet of potato chips and energy drinks. What he is still doing in this town, estranged from his parents, roaming about jobless and alone, is beyond me.

'My heart,' he moans.

As I take a history and connect the cardiac monitor, I relish this rare moment. Doesn't every son secretly dream of impressing his father with knowledge and skill? Our patient hardly requires expert emergency attention, but Dad observes my every move and his face is beaming.

Suspecting the patient has once again consumed too many Red Bulls, I offer him a trip to hospital and he nods. If I were him I too would rather spend my evening with the night-nurse than sit here alone. Once loaded up, I throw Dad the ambulance keys and give him a wink.

'Wanna drive? Someone's got to keep him company.'

For a second or two Dad stands there looking like a kid on Christmas morning.

No one visits me after that for the rest of my time in Peak Hill, but six months in I'm less concerned about isolation. Routines I've constructed help the time pass. I've also begun to feel the subtle tension that simmers below the surface of every country town, the whispering voices from unseen faces and the contradiction of personal privacy coupled with the compulsive curiosity to know the business of others. A lady in the grocery store last week was able to recite to me my every movement for three consecutive days: what time I left the station in the ambulance, where I drove to and what I did there. Sheep are dumb animals, she told me. My efforts to communicate with them at Jim Bolan's property were futile and stupid. I was speechless. Never on any visit to my fleecy friends had I seen another human being. Perhaps the sheep themselves were dobbing me in? Back in Sydney, where people live side by side and on top of one another, a person can saunter about naked in the backyard and no one pays the least bit of notice. Those who imagine they will find some kind of seclusion in a country retreat should think again.

It's August and my cases last month entailed an old man dead in his outhouse for at least a fortnight, a diabetic hypo to whom I administered Glucagon by subcutaneous injection and a motorcyclist with a broken femur on the road to Tullamore.

After browsing the internal vacancies around the state, I decide to apply for Hamilton in Newcastle. One of the controllers in Dubbo is a keen surfer like me and whenever he calls for a job we joke about starting a Western Division surfing team. I regret telling him about the Newcastle position because he immediately says he will go for it too, his length of service giving him a clear advantage.

As steady as I may be going in Peak Hill, the month ends with an accident that changes everything, an accident forcing me to leave town for my own safety.

At 10 pm on a Friday night I am in bed, lying awake in a silence one never hears in Sydney, imagining the wild time my friends are having there, bar-hopping around Darlinghurst and Surry Hills, seeing bands and DJs, laughing and flirting with girls.

When the phone rings, I jump back into the cold, dark room, sit bolt upright, snatching the receiver.

'Peak Hill Station.'

'Yeah mate, let's see ... some kid hit by a semi on the main street, says it's near the service station. I'll sort you out some back-up from Dubbo. They're just finishing a transfer so it might be an hour or so, maybe forty-five – if they fang it. Booked 10.01, on it 10.02. Good luck.'

No matter how many truck drivers Doug the policeman books for speeding through the main street, few semitrailers slow down much. They have a tight schedule and Peak Hill is just another blink-and-you-miss-it town clinging to the highway.

As it turns out, the fourteen-year-old Aboriginal boy lying in the gutter has only been 'clipped' by the semitrailer, a hit-and-run, although I suspect the driver wouldn't have noticed. A crowd from the mission has quickly formed and they urge me to hurry as I retrieve my gear.

'C'mon brudda, ya gotta help tha poor fella, he ain't in a good way mister medic.'

Relieved to find the boy conscious, I put him in a neck brace and begin a quick head-to-toe examination to ascertain his injuries. As I'm doing this I feel a hand squeeze my buttocks, more than one hand, in fact, until a good many are occupied with my bum cheeks. I look around but the crowd encircling me is too dense to identify a particular culprit. I wonder where Doug the policeman is, he always seems to arrive well after a drama is over.

The crowd shuffles back half a foot when I ask for some room, but pushes in again when I take a blood pressure reading. A second time I feel the hands, this time squeezing and caressing my buttocks with renewed enthusiasm, one of them even giving me an affectionate little slap. Such a thing is most distracting in emergency situations. Moreover, it's shameless sexual harassment. I grab my portable radio, calling for urgent police assistance. That should wake Doug up, I think to myself. Again I demand the onlookers move away, but my request is ignored.

'Listen brudda,' says an elder among the group. 'We don't trust you whitefellas, we gotta watch you, make sure you do us a good job, you know wad I mean?'

Finally Doug turns up, huffing and puffing and waving at the crowd to move on. Reluctantly they do, now giving me space to load the patient. Doug offers to drive the ambulance to the hospital and I call off my back-up from Dubbo as the boy seems to have suffered little more than minor abrasions.

Early the next morning I am woken by the sound of a car with holes in the muffler going up and down the dirt road beside the nurses' quarters. Crouching low, I crawl in my underwear to the kitchen where I'm able to peek out between the lace curtains on the window above the sink. Idling on the grass outside my place is a beaten-up, cream-coloured Datsun packed with Aboriginal girls.

'Shit,' I curse to myself. From my position at the window I can make out their conversation as they speculate on my whereabouts.

'He ain't come out from that house all morning, I reckon he in there, he in there, I'm telling ya.'

'Maybe he gone walkabout.'

'He ain't gone walkabout! Ambo guys don't go walkabout, they gotta be ready, you know, READY!'

'Yeah, and we seen two ambulance in that big shed, means he in there, he in there for sure!'

Not wanting to get caught undressed, I crab-crawl my way back to the bedroom and throw on my uniform, complete with all its formal trimmings. Maybe if I wear the tie and jacket with gold buttons down the front and speak with a firm tone I can scare off my stalkers. By the time I psych myself up to step out and challenge the girls – a butter knife in my pocket for reassurance – the Datsun does a donut, whipping up a cloud of dirt and farts off towards the highway. The girls catcall before the car shudders over the cattle grate at the end of the track and disappears.

I phone Doug and explain the situation.

'Yeah, I heard,' he says.

'Heard what?'

'The blackfellas are a bit upset with you.'

'Me? Why? I did fine with that kid last night.'

'Sure you did but you also got yourself a big problem in the process, mate. Those Koori chicks are trouble and you're the talk of the mission today. Heard they even got a special name for you, what is it again? Ah, Romeo! That's it!'

'Romeo?'

'Romeo, as in *Romeo and Juliet*, you know, that movie that's just come out?'

Baz Luhrmann's sexy contemporary interpretation of the Shakespearean classic had recently done good business at the Australian box office. Even Aboriginal kids in Peak Hill, miles from any cinema screen, knew about it. Unfortunately I didn't look anything like Leonardo DiCaprio. How could the girls have come to such a comparison based on the quality of my arse alone?

'Take it from me mate, whatever you do, don't be going down the mission on a job, understand? You'll either be set upon by the women or a jealous bloke will glass your throat.'

He paused for a moment. 'Actually, you got to get out of here. Those girls won't let up until they pin you down. Literally.'

'But Doug, you're a cop for crying out loud!'

'Come on. Cops can't touch no blackfella these days, let alone a female of the species. You know that. Sorry to tell you this, mate, you're on your own.'

Never have I covered the 20-metre distance between the nurses' quarters and the ambulance station in less time. Whatever door I pass through, I make certain it's bolted behind me. Despite Doug the policeman's fear-mongering, if a call comes in for the mission I have every intention of making an official request for his assistance. This way he cannot, by law, refuse to help me. The idea of driving anywhere near the southern part of town has put me on a knife's edge. What's to say a bitter indigenous bloke down there doesn't ring triple-0, fake some illness and jump up to strangle me with my own stethoscope?

My hopes of being nothing more than a passing interest are dashed the following day with the approach of the Datsun again at 10 am. It circles the ambulance station five or six times, coughing and backfiring. The car eventually skids to a stop and one of the girls gets out and peers through the window to see if I'm inside. Lying motionless behind the lounge, hiding for a good ten minutes, I wonder what my job has become. There is no question in my mind how different a situation like this would be if I were a female paramedic and my stalkers were male.

The *Bogan Times* comes out on Monday and 'Peak Hill's Romeo' is front-page news: 'Local Ambo Talk of the Town!'

Management in Dubbo are concerned. My wellbeing is under threat and the service has a responsibility for my safety next time there's a call to the Peak Hill mission.

Within a week I get surprising news. Out of all the applications for Hamilton Station, mine has been selected and I'm offered the position. With little hesitation I accept. Although I'm told the merit of my application won me the position, I'm unconvinced. My transfer takes effect immediately, which rarely happens. It seems obvious to me that the Newcastle job offer and my report of sexual harassment are no coincidence at all.

On the afternoon I get my transfer letter the Koori girls arrive again for their daily patrol. This time I lounge on the verandah in my underwear and give them a wave. Having eluded them for a fortnight, the girls scream in delight. A moment later the Datsun stalls and skids into a ditch. As the girl driving curses and tries starting it again, her accomplices lean out of the windows, yelling at the top of their voices.

'Hey, white boy!'

'Love your arse, white boy!'

'How about it, white boy!'

None of them actually leaves the car, and I sense for the first time they are too shy to come any closer.

'Love you, white boy!'

'Come and see us, white boy!'

Finally the engine splutters back to life. Before they pull onto the track again I make sure to blow them a kiss.

'Thank you, girls! Thank you!' I call after them.

The Datsun tumbles down and away in a flurry of hooting horns, wolf-whistles and flailing arms. When the dust settles and the road is quiet again, I'm overcome with shame for my unfounded anxieties. How harmless these girls were in reality, making the most of their life in this drab, nowhere town. A little innocent fun is all they ever wanted. Having finally lured the white boy medic from his house, I know in my heart they won't be back.

But neither will I.

RUNNING WITH THE LEOPARD

South Africa

Sleep will never visit me, lying on a paramedic's black leather lounge, imagining the lethal violence steaming across the city. Any moment now the phone will ring. My stomach is taut, turning with readiness, primed for action. Few men and women have slept, *truly* slept I mean, waiting for emergencies on a Jo'burg Friday night. Even Neil Rucker – The Leopard – is wide awake behind shut eyes.

A paramedic employed by Netcare 911, South Africa's second biggest ambulance service, The Leopard drives a late-model Audi and is permitted to work from home. The Leopard's modest red-brick house lies in a suburb close enough to the tough suburbs of Hillbrow and Berea for a quick response but far enough away to avoid bodies on his lawn in the morning.

'Like to be around my cats,' he says, pointing to a gallery of framed prints depicting handsome leopards crouching on the *veld*. Others recline on the boughs of trees yawning at sunset.

The Leopard's colleagues told me earlier in the day Rucker's nickname was inspired not only by his passion for the big cat, but his own cunning intelligence and skill, in particular his masterful intubation of patients with severe oropharyngeal trauma. He's got the veteran's look too – shaved head, a few good scars, eyes narrow and a little icy.

The Leopard lights some lotus incense with his Zippo and puts on a CD of meditation music. Slow synthesizers complement the sound of trickling from a water feature standing among indoor ferns. Despite the atmosphere of an Asian spa I still can't unwind. When the first call comes in I'm up like a jack-in-the-box.

Before we head off, The Leopard ducks into his bathroom and pulls the door shut. When he comes out he is wired-up, sniffing and rubbing his nose in the way a person would after snorting cocaine. I pretend not to notice. He may be suffering allergies, sinus problems.

'Here, put this on,' he says, passing me a bulletproof vest. It sits on my shoulders like a sack of rocks.

'Wow, it's heavy …'

'*Ja*, it's inlaid with ceramic. Don't worry, we won't be going swimming,' he says dryly.

The Leopard pops some chewing gum in his mouth, punches the air with his fists and grabs the car keys off the table. Seconds later we are rocketing along roads drenched in the apocalyptic orange light of street lamps, the engine of the Audi revving wildly, my body pushed back in the seat as The Leopard clocks 200 kilometres per hour into town.

Held over a week in a classroom at Witwatersrand – the university attached to Johannesburg General Hospital – the globally recognised Advanced Trauma Life Support (ATLS) course is meant to be intense. Conceived by the American College of Surgeons, in South Africa it is taught by those with perhaps the most experience in trauma anywhere in the world. Even with levels of violence in slow decline since the end of apartheid, Johannesburg makes no attempt to shake off its image as one of the most dangerous cities on earth. In 2008, *Time* magazine published figures showing an average of fifty-two murders occur in Johannesburg every twenty-four hours. This round-the-clock blunt and penetrating trauma ensures Jo'burg is to medics what Milan is to fashion designers. From Europe, Asia and the Middle East they come – doctors, nurses and paramedics – to learn the craft of saving lives in the 'golden hour' after severe physical damage to a human body from external forces.

Endotracheal intubation, decompression of tension pneumothoraces and cricothyroidotomies were all on the menu. I couldn't get enough of them. Many of the lectures and workshops practised skills beyond my previous level of training, skills I assumed to be out of my scope. Yet here I was, mixing it up with the best trauma surgeons in the world. I may have been transfixed by the experts, their stories and their tricks, yet had I known what the weekend would dish up on the streets of the capital, I would've been even more attentive.

After exiting The Leopard's responder I can barely stand up. My eyes sting from the acrid stench of his smoking brakes.

In the middle of the road, on a hill out of Berea, a man lies on his back gazing up at the starless night. Superstitious Good Samaritans have removed the victim's dirty *takkies*, placing the running shoes neatly beside his body, allowing a route of departure for his soul. Spreading from a single point on the man's parietal skull, a stream of bright red blood shimmers in our headlights, still flowing freely, finding new tributaries in the bitumen, branching out and joining up, coursing to an open drain.

The Leopard lights a cigarette and leans against the car.

I glance at him, then down at the man, then back again. 'Well?'

'Well, what?'

'He's breathing.'

'So? It's agonal. You wanna tube him? Here,' says The Leopard, casually opening the boot of the responder, retrieving his kit, passing it to me with his cigarette between his teeth, standing back again, entirely disinterested. Now that's burnout, I think to myself. Typical burnout. Speeding to the scene, then doing nothing.

'You won't do it?' I ask.

'He's chickenfeed, mate, all yours. Remember, don't pivot on the teeth. If there's blood in the airway, if you can't see the cords, forget about it. We're not going to stuff-up our suction this early in the shift.'

The vocal cords are Roman columns in the guy's throat and I sink the tube easier than expected. Once connected to a bag, I breathe him up. The Leopard steps on his cigarette. He slinks over swinging his stethoscope casually, pops it in his ears and listens over each side of the chest and once over the stomach. Without saying a word he nods his approval. From the leather pouch at his waist he whips out a pen torch, flicks it over the wounded man's eyes. The pupils are fixed on a middle distance, dilated to the edges, black as crude oil.

The Leopard chuckles.

'*Fok my*, do all you people come here for learning miracles? Makes me *lag*, eh.'

He points to my knees either side of the patient's head.

'By the way, you're kneeling in the brains.'

Early that morning I'd done a shift at Baragwaneth Hospital on the edge of Johannesburg's sprawling Soweto townships. With three thousand beds it is one of the largest hospitals in the world and treats more than two thousand patients a day. Half of these are thought to be HIV positive. A constant stream of ambulances unloaded their sorry cargo onto rickety steel beds lined up side by side until, by mid-afternoon, there was barely room for any more. Teamed up with Simon, an Australian doctor with whom I'd participated in the ATLS, we cannulated, medicated and sutured non-stop.

While joining a doctor's round in one of the wards, a boy of about sixteen was lying on a bed and as we passed by, he grabbed my wrist, pulling me close. His eyes pleaded as tears welled up and spilled onto his cheeks.

'Please, friend, take it out, please take it out.'

On his right chest I could see a small bulge, the shape of a bullet sitting just beneath the epidermis. Exit wounds are not always a given, I'd learnt.

'What's your name?'

'Treasure.'

'What happened to you?'

'Some men tried robbing me in Mofolo, I told them I had nothing to give but they *klapped* me hard and after I ran they shot.'

'Bastards. Did it enter your back?'

'*Ja*, bullet hit my spine, they told me it is shattered, they told me I am never walking again. When I fell down on the street I knew that. What will happen to me now? Last year my parents died in a minibus crash. There is no one to care for me.'

Already the doctors were three patients ahead – a ward round at Bara doesn't wait. Treasure squeezed my arm tighter, sensing my urge to move on.

'Please, brother, don't go, please, take it out.'

'Mate, I'm sorry for what happened to you, I really am. But the bullet is not interfering with any body function now, the damage is done. Maybe it will push out on its own one day.'

When I heard myself saying this to him – lying there unable to get up and walk to the open window, no father at the foot of his bed, no mother who named him her treasure holding his hand, no friends to help him pass the hours, the time he would forever spend turning over the memory of that one moment – I was filled with pity.

'Just want this evil thing out,' he said.

'One minute,' I told him. 'I'll bring a surgical kit.'

As I incised over the bullet, removing it with tweezers and dropping it into a steel kidney dish with a *clink*, I could feel Treasure's muscles relaxing under the drape. A deep sigh passed his lips and his face smoothed out with relief.

'God bless you, God bless you, God bless you,' he whispered with his eyes closed, as if I had just exorcised an evil spirit. 'God bless you forever.'

Among the pumps of a service station The Leopard unzips his bumbag. After looking around to make sure we are alone, he pulls out a 9mm semi-automatic handgun and slides out the magazine to show me its full load of rounds.

'Got another one strapped to my ankle,' he says.

With a sporadically effective police force, it is not unusual for paramedics to find themselves caught up in gunfights. Triage, the concept of sorting patients in multi-victim situations starting with the most critical, is superseded here by sheer self-preservation. If a member of one gang requests a paramedic to treat their own before those of an opposing group, it's usually at gunpoint. The Leopard takes no chances.

'Last year two of my colleagues were held up. Actually, it was an ambulance-jacking, they were left stranded in a bad place.'

As he drives me through Hillbrow, Johannesburg's most densely populated urban slum of decrepit high-rise buildings, I see a neighbourhood I wouldn't want to be stranded in either. Shopkeepers sit nervously behind thick iron bars and the blinking neon of pool halls and strip joints flickers on the figures of haggling prostitutes outside, their bodies shimmering with sweat.

'Some of us call it Hellbrow. New Year's Eve is the worst. People take pot shots with their guns from balconies, they let off fireworks horizontally, they throw furniture and other projectiles from windows, trying to hit people below. Few years back a fridge landed on a Metro ambulance. You never know what will come at you.'

Even ordinary party nights can be lethal in Jo'burg. Saturday evenings are difficult in most Western cities but here it's a warzone. Streets are jammed with people overflowing into the path of our car and the expectation of impending violence is palpable all around us. The Leopard locks the doors of the responder, says we'll avoid the worst parts of the suburb, places even he won't go unless accompanied by a police flying squad. He ignores red lights too, without being on a call. 'You've got to keep moving. Robots will kill you in Johannesburg,' he says, referring to the traffic signals. Rarely do I entertain irrational fears, but all heads seem turned on us tonight, eyes following the Audi as we pass, shady characters ready to pounce. In reality they could be just as well hoping we'll stop and join them for a drink, take a break, have a laugh. But as we draw level with the next pub where words stencilled by the door read 'No Guns Permitted', I'm not so sure.

'Zero Zero Three, come in.'

'Three, go ahead.'

'Man off a bridge, Yeoville.'

'Rrrroger.'

Tossing individuals off bridges and towering apartment buildings is a preferred method of murder for some gangs in Jo'burg. Without witnesses and no weapon or identifying wounds, these deaths can be easily mistaken for suicide.

As The Leopard does a U-turn he points to the tallest building in Hillbrow, the notorious Ponte City Apartment block. This cylindrical skyscraper with a hollow core was built in 1975 as a luxury condo fifty-four storeys high. After the end of apartheid many gangs moved in and the penthouse suite on the top floor became the headquarters of a powerful Nigerian drug lord.

'Once, we got half-a-dozen bodies in a week at the foot of that one,' he says, flicking on the siren. But this was 2003 and things were changing. Using the South African Army as back-up, developers were evicting undesirables. Whether Ponte City's former glory can be restored remains to be seen. Selling luxury apartments in the heart of a suburb where visiting the corner store for a carton of milk can get you killed will be tricky.

Half a minute down the road in Yeoville the traffic is backed up and we use the breakdown lane, our red and blue lights bouncing off the vehicles we pass. Under a freeway overpass we pull up behind a police van and see the officer in lane two standing over a young man lying face down, illuminated by the headlights of a late model Mercedes.

'Lucky he missed the poor lady's car, nice Merc that one,' jokes the policeman. A woman in the front seat dabs her cheeks with a tissue.

I look up. The overpass is a good 20 or 25 metres high. No wonder the patient is groaning in agony. I'm surprised he's even conscious.

Behind me The Leopard approaches with our gear. Seems the case has inspired him to show me what he's made of. Or maybe the siren of our back-up ambulance wailing towards us has compelled him to act.

The policeman helps by manually stabilising the patient's head. Calmly the Leopard scissors off the man's shorts and T-shirt to expose him for a better examination. He slips a wide-bore IV into the *cubital fossa* without blinking and throws me a bag of Hartmann's solution.

'Five minutes on scene or we get docked,' scoffs The Leopard. 'Patient's got an open-book pelvis with jelly legs, but it's all about those five bloody minutes.' He shakes his head and I know what he means. Time to hospital is the essence in trauma, but proper immobilisation, effective analgesia, cautious extrication and transport strategies will all, in the long run, reduce morbidity. Only by working the road can one truly appreciate 'time' as but one factor among many upon which an ambulance service should be judged.

Once the line is clear of air I connect and open it for a bolus. The Leopard double-checks the blood pressure, palpating seventy systolic. Falls from great heights often cause serious pelvic fractures like this, lacerating vessels internally and resulting in massive blood loss filling body cavities. This, in turn, can lead to absolute hypovolaemia – a condition of low blood volume – that could prove fatal.

'Keep the fluids going wide open, we'll shut it off at ninety systolic. Don't go over ninety, got it?'

I nod.

Three paramedics from a Basic Life Support (BLS) ambulance arrive. They too comment on how lucky it is the Mercedes escaped damage. Two of them help with patient care, while the third, a stern-looking African man with spectacles on the end of his nose and epaulettes studded with shiny stars, stands to one side and starts a stopwatch hanging round his neck.

The Leopard looks over at me and rolls his eyes. 'What did I tell you? Five minutes, let's go!' Maybe The Leopard is burnt out but tonight he's playing the game. We're being timed like athletes, timed by a stoney-faced supervisor with a digital stopwatch. Crazy.

Medics from the ambulance drag over a flat spine-board onto which we lay some pelvic sheeting. Once the patient is rolled over, we use this to stabilise him from the waist down, wrapped and clamped. Any unnecessary movement in pelvic fractures, even multiple examinations springing the iliac crests, increases internal bleeding and risk of death.

'One, two, three, lift!' The stretcher legs lock down and the trolley is wheeled to the ambulance. As the supervisor gets in the front seat he glances over at us and laughs.

'Hey Rucker, four minutes, thirty-three. Close shave!'

The Leopard grunts and lights a cigarette.

From Netcare's depot at Milpark we watch a retrieval helicopter descend onto a landing pad at the doorstep of the company's very own fully equipped trauma hospital.

'Heard it on the radio,' The Leopard tells me. 'Some lion safari gone wrong, a 4x4 rollover.'

Running parallel to public medical services, Netcare has fifty-three private hospitals like this throughout South Africa and Swaziland. Milpark alone employs some of the country's brightest doctors, offering every imaginable specialty and a staggering ninety intensive care beds. For those who can afford private health cover the company has become South Africa's provider of choice. But as an act of goodwill to the poorer people of South Africa, Netcare offers its ambulance services free to those who earn below a certain income threshold. Nowadays, the vast majority of emergency calls are made by non-subscribers. These patients are, however, always conveyed to public hospitals. Although it is currently common practice in South Africa to dial 911 – Netcare's clever exploitation of the widely known US emergency number – bystanders will also ring the government's metro ambulance service at the same time. In a crisis people will take whatever ambulance comes first.

As a consequence, driving to emergencies has become a frantic race between the public and private services. This 'healthy competition' has only improved response times in Johannesburg, according to Netcare medics. Relationships between crews from both systems generally remain harmonious despite this challenge. Stress comes instead from pressure placed on them by management to reach the scene first in order to uphold the service's image as the quickest.

While good for the public, it's a dangerous game for medics. In 2002, nineteen ambulances were written-off in the city of Johannesburg, mostly by Metro Ambulance Service drivers. Netcare are not so worried. Official figures show their average response times are five minutes faster than the government service.

'Sometimes on the way to hospital with the patient we pass the Metro ambulance still heading to the scene,' chuckles The Leopard. 'We always give a little wave, of course.'

As we prowl for work in those raw, bloodstained streets of central Johannesburg, I have become The Leopard's cub, learning to hunt with the master.

'Are you ever afraid?' I ask him. Stories of gun battles with drug gangs, resuscitations at knifepoint and snipers taking shots at reflective vests have kept me on the edge of my seat all night.

'*Ja*, sure I get afraid.'

'Of what?'

'HIV.'

It isn't what I expected him to say.

'Average sixty people are shot every day here, ten thousand people die on the roads each year, 90 per cent of our calls are trauma, but HIV is the leading cause of death. At least 20 per cent of sub-Saharan Africa is HIV positive. Just do the math. If you consider 90 per cent of our work is trauma with active bleeding and 20 per cent of these patients are HIV positive, you will understand what we're really afraid of. Get blood on you in Australia, England, America and you don't sweat much. Get blood on you here and you don't sleep till the results come back.'

The Leopard plans to enrol in a paramedic research degree, a doctorate perhaps. 'I need to get off the road. I have children now, they live with my wife but I want to see more of them. You know,

I have a responsibility to them, a responsibility to stay alive.'

The streets of Johannesburg seem eons away from the immense beauty of South Africa's wilderness. The contrast is extreme. But then, some of the most stunning places in the world have a dark underbelly, a place shared by the poor, the sad, the criminal, the beggar, the victim and the paramedic.

'Zero zero three?'

Reluctantly The Leopard picks up the handset and replies. Our lights and siren ignite the dark road ahead.

'It's not a bad neighbourhood, this,' says The Leopard. 'We're less than a kilometre from Hillbrow, I have a drink here sometimes, you know, during the daytime.'

But descending a steep hill we are first on the scene of a chaos like none I've encountered.

From what I can make out, a fully laden semitrailer lost control, veered to the opposite side of the road, crushed five cars and continued on to plough through a restaurant packed with diners, finally coming to rest deep within the building.

The carnage is widespread and horrific.

Bodies lie everywhere. Cries and screams and groans puncture the air. Hands pull us this way and that. I'm dizzy and cannot focus on any one patient, there are so many, perhaps twenty, perhaps more. Where do we start? Triage, triage. My French comes back to me. We need to sort them, make sense of it, get perspective.

The Leopard is so cool it shames me. He strides through the devastation like a war-hardened general, calmly slipping his hands into latex gloves. He takes no gear, no oxygen kit, no medicine, no bandages. Just the man and his portable radio. One at a time he stoops down to check the breathing and circulation of those lying motionless. Effortlessly he elicits responses from those who are conscious and checks the smashed vehicles and the truck for occupants. As I follow behind him, I finally hear him speak into his handset, his voice steady and commanding, his report plain and precise.

'MVA, truck versus restaurant, no persons trapped, four dead, sixteen patients on the ground, unknown number of walking wounded, need fire brigade and as many ambulances you've got handy.'

The Leopard grabs my shoulder and points to a man lying near a car that looks like it's been through a wrecking yard. 'Start with that guy, he's not well. I'm going to delegate the back-up as it comes.'

From the responder I get our gear and race back, stepping over the bodies of those beyond help.

'He can't feel his legs,' cries the man's wife, crouching beside him. 'He can't feel them!'

I ask her name. It's Melanie. She tells me the patient is Martin. Today is their wedding anniversary and he took her for dinner, alfresco, with candles.

'Listen,' I grab her attention. 'Melanie, you've got to help me now. Here, take Martin's head and don't let it move. Keep talking to him. Stay calm because you need to keep *him* calm. We've got a job to do and we'll do the job together.'

After fitting the oxygen mask, I mould a hard collar round Martin's neck and begin a head-to-toe examination. His breathing is rapid and shallow. I place my stethoscope in his armpits and listen. Limited air entry on the right, I'm certain of it. There is movement and crepitus, a popping sound and grating of crushed ribs when I palpate the chest wall. I suspect a collapsed lung. It may be tensioning, in which case an immediate procedure to release the pressure with a needle is required. As I break out in a sweat at the prospect of doing this, a Netcare ambulance team with a senior paramedic join me and begin cannulating and getting ready to board the patient. They will decompress the man's chest once loaded up, the medic tells me. They work at lightning speed and I wonder if another supervisor is standing somewhere in the shadows holding a stopwatch.

Medics are swarming all over the site now. Metro EMS, Netcare 911, even ER24, a company I've not yet come across. Suddenly The Leopard is behind me, leaning in.

'*Boet*,' he says in Afrikaans, meaning 'brother'. 'We got to go, we got a gunshot to the head just round the corner, they got no one for it.'

I'm stunned. Broken glass crunches and mixes with blood underfoot as I carry the responder kit back to the car. It's an awkward response in tragic times, but as I get into the front seat I begin to laugh. I laugh at the sheer absurdity of leaving the biggest accident of my career to attend a shooting. I laugh because it has taken me less than twenty-four hours to reach this point, this point where a paramedic's work in Johannesburg is encapsulated entirely by a single, staggering moment of madness.

And the night is but young.

SHEIK, RATTLE AND ROLL

England

On the rain-drenched morning Henry takes the wheel I am secretly relieved the old man we are carting from one sad nursing home to another is afflicted by a state of dementia so advanced he is seemingly oblivious to our existence and stares silently ahead into a land beyond. Normally I wouldn't wish the illness on my worst enemy. But as Henry pushes the siren and races down Herne Hill towards Brixton at the speed of a Grand Prix driver on amphetamines, it's a good thing our patient – someone's dear grandpa – is numb to it all. The old man bounces around like a leg of ham in a delivery van. In fact, groceries and daily mail probably get better rides than this in London.

Approaching the intersection of Milkwood Road and Half Moon Lane is where we have the fourth near miss of the day. A car appears from nowhere, as Henry puts it afterwards, making it sound like a supernatural phenomenon beyond human comprehension. While hurtling through the red signal without slowing I assume this apparition has approached from the right, but I see nothing at all as I'm riding in the back clutching a crossbar with one hand and the patient's shoulder with the other. When Henry plants his generous weight on the brakes I'm only half ready for it. Equipment flies into the front cabin, some of it catching me while passing. Airborne oxygen masks and kidney dishes are the least of my concerns. Our old man, drooling and wide-eyed, has long lost the instinct to hold onto the stretcher rails and our extreme deceleration threatens to catapult him through the windscreen. I have little choice but to throw myself on top of the patient, his brittle bones digging into me as I pin him to the mattress with my body. A sound of screeching tyres and angry horns is followed by the choking smoke of burning rubber pumping into the back of the wagon.

'You all right, geezer?' Henry asks once he has pulled over past the intersection, his face pale and puffing.

'Think so,' I say in a neutral tone, until it occurs to me how pissed-off I really am and I add, 'Why the urgency anyway, mate? We're going to a bloody nursing home.'

'He should 'ave seen me comin', tha bastard.'

But Henry has only himself to blame and he knows it. Lights and sirens are merely a *request* for people to give way, not a demand.

Henry's hands are trembling as he collects the bits and pieces littering the front cabin. Though he seems shaken, I know he will do it again, maybe even today. Like a poker machine that eventually pays out, we're long overdue for a prang. And if eventually he kills a man, or more than one, I want nothing to do with it.

Got to quit, got to quit, got to quit.

What am I still doing here?

With its prestigious-sounding name no one would suspect a shoddy operation from this private Harley Street ambulance service. Ambulances plush as limousines, I thought. Only these would satisfy the British high society and foreign millionaires who visit the nation's famous strip of specialist rooms and luxury clinics.

Perhaps the greatest insult one can give a genuine paramedic is to call him or her an ambulance driver, yet this is what I was, my paramedic degree as useful as a sheet of toilet paper. The art of driving grannies to doctors' appointments had, as I recall, never been covered. Why my skills were unattractive to the London Ambulance Service (LAS) when I applied for recognition of prior learning, I just don't know. The LAS was naturally my first choice, but the process facing foreign paramedics hoping to get on London's ambulances is known to be so long and painful that most don't bother. Ironically, ambulance services in sunnier countries of the world like Australia and New Zealand have made quite a business of poaching British paramedics and have done this so aggressively over the past decade it has created a shortage of paramedics in England, and a minor political storm.

Wasted skills aside, better money can be made working for private patient transport services anyway, even if it represents a significant drop in action. Nor is it wise to remain jobless while waiting for the bureaucratic process of the National Health Service. As Iraqi doctors and Iranian surgeons flipping burgers in London's takeaway joints can attest, survival rules over pride in this cruellest of cities. Yes, we'd all like to work in our chosen careers, but decent heating and square meals are the only way to get through winter, and Kass, my then girlfriend now wife, needs a new woollen coat. Still, I wish we had chosen Barcelona over London when deciding on a city in which to base ourselves for a few years of European exploration.

It's colder than deep-sea diving off Alaska. Even with the windows up and my green fleece zipped tight I feel like an ice sculpture. We drop the patient off at his five-star nursing home – quite literally 'drop' as Henry claims he 'wasn't ready' with the head end of the stretcher at the moment I called 'one, two, three'. I've come to expect this kind of thing when Henry is way past his fried chicken and chips time. It will be his third lot in a single morning. Another of his shirt buttons is sure to pop before the day's end.

We park at a Harley Street corner so we can make a rapid response to the next boring transfer. As the rain thunders on the window, I watch Henry munching fried chicken, getting it tangled in his scraggly ginger beard and dropping it down the front of his uniform. In fact, his uniform is already stained from previous fried chickens. With a belly like that there's only one place falling chicken tends to land.

'So, you is telling me you once got a hundred quid tip off a Arab?' he says as he eats, displaying the contents of his mouth.

'Yeah, Kuwaiti royal family.'

'Kuwai-i royal family?' he licks his lips, looks annoyed. 'I neva got nufink offa tha Kuwai-i royal family. Took one of 'em in too, I did. Had a hip done, he did. But tha Kuwai-i royal family never looked arfta Henry, did vey.'

I sigh and glance at my watch, wondering what the Kuwaiti royal family would have thought about an ambulance stinking of fried chicken, driven by a maniac.

'Mate, you know we got a Arab later on,' says Henry, 'four-firtey in from Heafrow …'

'*An* Arab, Henry, it's *an* Arab.'

'Yeah, dats wot I said, a *Arab*.'

Worst thing about having an ambulance with a broken stereo is that it forces one to listen to a partner chewing fried chicken and using bad English in England.

'Well,' I reply, 'it's nearly two o'clock, and you know the traffic.'

Henry knows the traffic all right. This is part of the problem. He loves nothing more than to plan his day so that unless we use our lights and sirens we'll be late to every appointment and pick-up. This is because, quite frankly, he loves to use the lights and sirens. When I first met Henry I spotted him right away as a wannabe paramedic who never made the grade. Being an ambulance driver is a little boy's fantasy as much as being a train driver or bus driver. In most emergency medical systems, however, ambulance drivers must also use clinical skills normally reserved for doctors. This naturally excludes a good number of candidates, Henry included. Society is full of disappointed men and women who have longed to drive ambulances from the age of five when they spent each day constructing matchbox car crashes and sending matchbox ambulances to the scene. Recruitment departments of public emergency services are perpetually inundated by such applicants and spend half their time palming them off.

The only other qualified paramedic working at the company was fired from the London Ambulance Service for visiting a Kensington barbershop while on duty. When I heard this I told him it sounded like unfair dismissal. Medics are normally permitted to visit coffee houses and corner stores in their catchments so long as they can quickly respond. Why not a barbershop? I mean, how long does it take to throw off an apron, brush down a uniform and go out with half a cut? Not long at all. If anything, the gentleman's commitment to looking sharp and tidy in the workplace should have been commended. As much as I'd prefer it I'm never assigned to work with him. Our boss wants one qualified medic per wagon. And apart from the two of us, the rest are a bunch of fantasists who recently discovered a community college somewhere outside London conducting a five-day first-aid course they believe allows them to use the title 'paramedic'. Never mind it took me four years of study to earn the same. While I don't bother wearing anything at all to identify myself as one, these men could not be more decorated. From emergency service catalogues they have mail-ordered paramedic insignia of every description. Cloth patches, embroidered epaulettes, shiny badges, clip-on pins, reflective vests and so on, all emblazoned with the word 'paramedic'; one ambulance driver is so covered in pins and badges he looks like a walking Christmas tree.

Then there is the gear. While I have trouble locating my stethoscope most days, these men have got every imaginable utility dangling from their belts. There are Leatherman knives, wallets for gloves and scissors, phone holders, torches of various sizes, rolls of Leucoplast, radio holsters, mini disinfectant dispensers, rubber tourniquets and various other oddly-shaped black pouches containing everything but handcuffs. All these are attached for the prime purpose of looking as much like a paramedic as possible, or at least how they *imagine* a paramedic must look. This I find most entertaining and wonder how I've managed to do the same job for so long with nothing on my belt but a buckle.

While some veteran medics would be irritated by such things, I am way more frustrated by the widespread and reckless use of emergency warning devices.

Prince Abdullah al-Sabah's private jet is to land at Heathrow in twenty minutes and, as I remember from my last conversation with an al-Sabah, they are not fond of tardiness. The Sabahs are thought to hold the largest number of shares in almost all blue-chip companies in the Western world and to have a combined family wealth of US$200 billion. On first meeting the Kuwaitis, my politeness to a veiled female family member was generously rewarded with a crisp fifty pound note pulled from a wad of cash thick as a brick and dispensed by a *keffiyeh*-wearing aide. Accepting money from patients beyond the agreed payment for services is considered unethical in the medical profession and strictly forbidden for government ambulance workers and hospital staff. But in London's private health care, tipping seems somehow acceptable and is not uncommon.

'White car on the left!' I warn Henry as he comes dangerously close to clipping a sedan that has failed to pull over far enough.

My head is throbbing with the beat of the siren. The Ford Transit parts traffic out of the city like Moses did the Red Sea. It's slow going, but we're getting through faster than anyone else.

What is the public thinking, I wonder, those distressed commuters struggling to edge out of our way, imagining the worst? What if they knew that Henry was using his lights and sirens because he thinks it's fun, because he intentionally ate his fried chicken slow enough for the traffic to build up? And what if they knew I was letting him do it because I'd hate to be late for the Kuwaiti royal family, because I'm hoping for another tip, more than last time – if I'm lucky.

Back in Sydney severe consequences result from the inappropriate use of lights and sirens. Not that we'd bother, anyway. We're so busy most of the time it's a relief when the siren is off, allowing us a little peace and quiet. Warning devices are only a novelty for those who don't use them much.

'Ow of tha way! Comin' fru! Move it! Move it! Move it!' shouts Henry.

'They can't hear you,' I say, wishing he'd shut up.

'All right, but vey can *see* me, can't vey.'

'See you what?'

'See me yellin'. Yellin' and gesticalatin'!'

I don't know how many private ambulance services there are in London, but ever since routine patient transport was outsourced, every little boy rejected from the LAS could finally drive an ambulance as fast as they like with 'blues and twos' – blue flashing lights and a two-tone siren. It was absurd and out of control. By my second day at this company I'd survived three near-death experiences and one flying patient. But when I raised the matter with the boss – a middle-aged, chain-smoking, sarcastic woman with the face of an East London gangster – she looked me square in the eye and croaked, 'You know by now what the traffic in London is like, son, don't you?'

And I replied, 'Yes, but it's dangerous going fast without a pressing reason.'

And she said, 'Harley Street patients are special, you understand. They expect the best. They have never waited for anything in their lives. They don't expect to lie in ambulances while our drivers inch along in traffic, do they now?'

But a day later she inadvertently revealed her true reason for ignoring the fun crews were having with lights and sirens when Henry called up and told her we were unlikely to complete two jobs in the designated time frame.

'Well,' she said via the crackly radio, 'what have you got those pretty lights on your wagon for, Henry?'

Turnover. It is all about turnover and profit. The faster we do a job, the quicker we're on to the next. We make deliveries like any courier company, but because we deliver human cargo we can make our deliveries in half the time by halting on-coming traffic and momentarily paralysing city intersections.

Henry brakes heavily. 'Wanka!' he shouts.'Got evry fink on, idiot!'

And with everything on we skid into Heathrow making such a racket that for a second airport security must think some hijacking has taken place without their knowledge.

But no, all this Arab wants is a quality heart bypass.

We meet the patient sunk into a deep leather recliner in the lavish corporate jet building, a man in his sixties wearing a stiff white *dishdasha* and rockstar sunglasses. He's very pleased when I greet him with the traditional *Assalam Aleikum* but looks with a little disgust at Henry who struggles to negotiate a leather ottoman with the stretcher.

'How was your flight?' I ask the sheik.

'*Bekhair*,' he says, and his aide appears, a different one from last time, and translates.

'Fine, he says flight is fine, thank you,' says the aide.

Henry is by my side now. I can smell him.

'Good to go ven?' he asks, looking at the aide expectantly. But no wad of cash appears and we stand in awkward silence, a silence like the one after hotel porters take your bags up and you don't have any change to tip them with. Why Henry expects the sheik will slip him some cash *before* he's been driven anywhere is beyond me.

After half a minute, Henry readies the stretcher and we help the sheik climb on.

It's a rough ride back to Harley Street. I've strapped the sheik down well but notice the skin over his knuckles blanche while gripping the stretcher rails. The sheik says something loudly to his aide, raising his voice over Henry's siren. I fear that any chance of getting a tip now is out of the question. But I'm wrong. Instead of lodging his complaint about the journey, the sheik's aide leans over and thrusts a fifty pound note into my palm.

'No, no, I'm not supposed to take this,' I protest.

But Henry's siren is so loud I can't really hear myself and when I try to hand the money back the sheik's aide takes it and forcefully stuffs it into my top pocket. There is a certain desperation in the way he has given me the tip that makes me think for a moment I'm being bribed to take the wheel and slow things down. When Henry veers sharply to avoid something and leans on the horn for thirty seconds, cursing grotesquely, I consider it. In Kuwait, my partner would be promptly executed for driving like this with an al-Sabah on board. *'Allah, Allah, Allah!'* cries the sheik.

Really got to quit, I think. The fifty pounds in my top pocket will hardly tide me over until the next job. But I don't care.

After dropping off the sheik at a cardiologist, Henry curses the Kuwaiti royal family for not helping us out and how the House of Saud is far more generous.

I shrug, choosing not to mention my tip.

'Henry,' I say politely as we reach the Baker Street tube station, 'you don't mind dropping me off here, do you?'

'Right 'ere?' he asks, raising his eyebrows.

'Yes please. And do me another favour, will you?'

'What's tha'?'

'Tell the boss I've resigned.'

ALL QUIET! NEWS BULLETIN!

The Philippines

Lumbering like the giant propellers of an ocean liner, the fan blades turn too slowly and too high above us to cool the night. But the loose chugging and whooshing is sending me to sleep. Behind a heavy wooden desk illuminated by a strip of neon screwed into one of the peppermint-green walls is the chief of the Philippine General Hospital's Emergency Medical Service, Manolo Pe-Yan, a plump man, unusually serious for a Filipino. Seriousness, however, does not always translate to professional appearance and Manolo is wearing the same singlet he's been wearing for a week, stained by a dark bib of sweat, his head tipping forward then up again as he sleeps.

It's 1 am on a Saturday morning. Two white uniform shirts are hanging on the posts of a single steel bed beside me. Snoring soundly upon it, curled up together despite the heat, is a crew of emergency medical technicians (EMTs) seemingly content with the status quo – a parked ambulance and no calls on a night when all manner of accidents and murders are occurring in the action-packed metropolis. A stone's throw from where these medics are sleeping there is a constant stream of jeepneys, taxis and tricycles screeching to a halt outside the hospital emergency department. Onto the doorstep their contents are dumped: an assortment of stabbed and mauled victims; unconscious men with occluded airways, bodies made limp by the fractures of long falls and pedestrians with broken necks. Last week I worked a few shifts in the emergency department and dragged these people in, seeing how nasty and critical injuries and medical cases become without pre-hospital care. And while I did this, across an island of lawn and flowerbeds, under a low tin awning, two beautiful late-model Chevrolet ambulances stood washed and polished – and silent.

'Okay, *tayo marinig ng ibang* song!' Another Filipino hit is announced on a little transistor radio. It's all we listen to. A World War II ceiling fan and cheesy music, neither of which is ever switched off – the ceiling fan for obvious reasons and the radio because, in its truest definition relating to ambulance work, we are listening out for jobs. There is still no central emergency number in The Philippines, no control room or ambulance dispatch. So we wait, as we do most days and nights, monitoring the half-hour news bulletins on ordinary FM radio and the occasional updates between Pinoy rock classics by Sugar Hiccup and Tropical Depression. Occasionally, maybe once a week, a member of the public will arrive breathless at the ambulance station, pointing in the general direction of some traffic collision nearby. But mostly we wait for a radio announcement – sometimes for weeks on end – about a pile-up on one of the many highways and skyways crossing Manila. Last month, both ambulance crews took it upon themselves to respond to a train derailment after hearing a report on the radio, but have since done little else.

The air is thick with humidity and the smell of green mangoes. I look around the room and see I'm the last one awake. Having no comprehension of Tagalog, the 1 am news means nothing to me. Half of Manila may have gone up in flames and I wouldn't know. Nor would my colleagues stir from their slumber. There is nothing to do but stretch out on a bench near the door and submit to the urge to close my eyes.

In heat like this my dreams are always bizarre. The emperor of a mighty country, suddenly inspired into a random act of generosity, orders all hungry tramps in the land to be issued a jar of his finest caviar. But one of the tramps is unhappy and says, 'Just give me a damn sandwich!' The tramp says this about the same time I wake up and turn over. While I drift off to sleep again I comprehend the dream may well have been about our two ambulances donated by the United States government. They came with the latest, high-tech equipment, with pulse oximetry, twelve-lead ECG machines and pneumatic ventilators. Like caviar to a tramp are these ambulances to The Philippines' largest public hospital. Only yesterday we took a patient in from another facility hooked up to our automatic ventilator and found there were *no* ventilators in the intensive care unit of the hospital. How odd it was to see our state-of-the-art device replaced by a simple bag-valve-mask – a bag manually squeezed every four seconds or so by the patient's beloved without interruption, sometimes for months. No wonder the bag-valve-mask is known here as as a 'relative ventilator'. And because the chain of health care is only as strong as its weakest link, there was considerable discussion among the EMTs about why they bothered connecting the ventilator in the first place. More interesting to me was to volunteer in a country where ambulances are better equipped than the hospitals they deliver to. It's May 1998 and I'm only here for six weeks – half my time ambulance-riding, half island-hopping – far too short a period to help create awareness of a paramedical service among twenty million people in the most densely populated city in the world.

Manolo nudges me with a Philippine breakfast plate of *champorado* – a combination of sticky chocolate rice served with salty fish, a fish which I detest and usually discreetly dispose of so as not to offend my hosts.

'We have very important meeting in the evening, Joe,' grunts Manolo, using the rather annoying nickname I share with every other Western male who bears the slightest resemblance to an American GI. Manolo's face doesn't give anything away, even when I know he's being funny. I'm certain it's his own type of humour, that he's one of those straight-faced funny men.

I raise my eyebrows and take the bowl.

'Chinese Fire Brigade again?' I ask.

'You'll see, Joe,' he answers.

The two EMTs, Juan and Fermin, are awake. Fermin is brushing his teeth in a sink by the door while Juan runs a comb through his hair over and over again, staring ahead with a drowsy gaze. Neither of them bothers getting into their uniform shirts. They only do this if a job comes in or while escorting me across town to the headquarters of the Chinese Fire Brigade where I lecture in first aid. Three nights ago they also turned out nicely for a dinner with the fire chief whose selection of deep-fried insects and marinated grubs revolved on the centre of the table like a carousel of horrors. With this grisly platter still in mind, I hope this evening's meeting will be nowhere near Chinatown.

Manolo snaps at Fermin to turn off the tap.

'All quiet! News bulletin!' he barks.

Roadworks have begun on a new flyover and taxes will go up for a year to pay for it. Joseph Estrada, one of the country's most popular film stars, is running for the next election and looks likely to win it. The temperature is 36 degrees Celsius with 98 per cent humidity. Heavy showers are predicted for later in the afternoon. And Silvana cookies – according to a radio promotion – now come in the flavours of coconut and purple yam. That's all. No bus accidents, ongoing hostage situations, no gangland massacres or people threatening to jump off buildings.

With nothing better to do we mop the ambulance for the tenth time in a week. Considerably more mopping goes on here than any treatment of patients. Mopping detergent with detergent, as Juan always says. Oxygen we check too, and not because it is used for patients short of breath, but for the chance that a slow leak may have dropped the levels. This is the life of a public ambulance service medic in Manila – mopping, cleaning, sleeping …

And waiting for news bulletins.

Our meeting after work, as it turns out, is merely a visit by the rest of the station staff, three of them in all, who, out of pure sympathy for the boredom suffered by their colleagues on shift, have come to bring us a hot dinner. Sunny – a young EMT behind The Philippines Emergency Medical Technician's Association (PEMTA), which presently boasts a total of seven members – lugs in a small television set and box of cables. He connects them up and tests a microphone with a crackly 'one, two, two!' Moments later we are sitting round drinking San Miguel beer, singing karaoke.

'You have choice,' says Sunny when it is my turn with the microphone. "New York, New York" or "Barbie World".

Great! Cringing, I tell Sunny these are not the most interesting songs but see few alternatives in the open catalogue. Reluctantly, I ask him to start the Sinatra.

To my great relief, after just one 'New York' into the song, Manolo interrupts.

'All quiet!' he yells. 'News bulletin!'

DR AQUARIUS
AND THE GYPSIES

Macedonia

Saints are always good for a holiday. A couple of weeks ago it was Saint George and, now, in the middle of a Balkan summer, it's Saint Nicholas who really ought to be celebrated at Christmas. But who cares if they want to honour him twice? It's an excuse for a party and the fact that I'm working all weekend is no obstacle. Not in Macedonia, not among the doctors and nurses and drivers of Skopje 194.

Along the potholed road into the city, looking out from the peeled tinting of the side window, I catch glimpses of grubby youths half-heartedly kicking footballs in overgrown parks under the bleak housing blocks where they live. None of them waves at the ambulance as kids always do back home, hoping for a blast from our siren. On benches, watching them play, stumpy old men sit with motionless wives, saying nothing. At a corner where we pause for a red light a little boy sells eggs from a tray. A gypsy girl does a half-hearted tap dance in front of cars and someone throws her a coin. Homeless dogs scratch themselves in the heat. At a nearby kiosk with torn beach umbrellas outside, a row of bicycles lean against a sun-cracked wall. Behind that, the spire of a mosque rises between apartment blocks where laundry flaps from narrow windows. Here the best suburbs can look like decrepit public housing estates. Like my parents' photographs from their European travels in the 1970s, everything seems faded and bathed in a vinegary orange light, as if one is moving through an era long passed.

Skopje is littered with the evidence of better times. This city was a base for Alexander the Great, the birthplace of Mother Teresa, the place made beautiful in the Byzantine era and under the Ottomans. It was still beautiful on the day before the earthquake of 1963 when 90 per cent of the city was flattened. Rebuilt by Yugoslavs with a concrete obsession, Skopje became something else and then, when communist rule ended between 1990 and 1992 (and Yugoslavia broke up with Macedonia claiming independence in 1991), the money for public works dried up. Once grand fountains ceased their squirting but still remain as concrete eyesores in every empty plaza. City gardens are knee-high in grass and weeds, pavements are fractured or caved in completely and a whimsical Socialist-era fun park on the edge of town has not changed in forty years. As for the Macedonian dress sense, everyone appears to be clothed in drab and mismatched garments they have quite conceivably selected from suburban charity shops while blindfolded.

Three months earlier in Sydney, my paramedic partner and I were called to a woman originally from Macedonia now living in a small flat crammed with imposing floral lounges, a woman who felt the need to phone our emergency ambulance for what she described as a 'burning tongue'. There is, of course, no documented protocol for such a complaint, but as far as we could gather her tongue was not alight, nor did it look particularly red or swollen or suffering the effects of hot curry or chilli pepper or any other such thing. What we did observe about her, however, was a level of nervous tension that commonly precedes inexplicable symptoms like this and is more often related to mental rather than physical origins.

As a lover of Balkan music I knew a little about the Roma gypsies residing in Eastern Europe, many in the small country of Macedonia, a country of just two million people, landlocked by Greece, Bulgaria, Serbia and Albania. What I didn't know was that Macedonia is also host to the largest community of gypsies in the world, most of them living in a ghetto – or *maalo* – known as Shutka.

After the burning tongue I got to thinking about where on earth it might be appropriate to call ambulances for such a complaint. And although people call for some pretty interesting things just about everywhere, my mind persistently returned to Macedonia. Eager to explore not only the blood-and-guts of my industry but the varying cultural peculiarities that affect it, I booked a ticket.

There are two reasons why Macedonian ambulances are always snug in the front seat. Firstly, both doctor and nurse sit beside the driver. That's three in a row. Secondly, most medics at Skopje 194 have a considerable girth, for which the Macedonian diet is clearly to blame. Here, a meal without yellow cheese is considered inedible, even fresh salad is topped with it. Nevertheless, winters in Skopje can be nasty and the cuddly warmth of a colleague is always welcome.

While all the drivers are male, most of the doctors and nurses are not. Unlike many ambulance services that struggle to attract female recruits, in Macedonia ladies run the entire show. Dr Maja Poposka, the surprisingly young and attractive director of the service is fond of black power suits and high heels, and is a stark contrast to the legion of women she commands who mostly have the attitude and build of lady prison guards. Even in their white scrubs, wooden clogs and dainty black doctor bags, these women could suffocate the toughest male paramedic in their fathomless bosoms. They bark at their patients in voices deepened by Marlboro Reds and give every physical indication that they mean business.

For the weekend of the 2010 Saint Nicholas holiday I have submitted to being the plaything of a lively lady doctor with a black beehive and cherry-red lipstick. She is known simply as Dr Aquarius and she calls me Benja. Dr Aquarius is assisted by a nurse named Snezhana Spazovska who has several sparkling diamantes set in her front teeth and painted fingernails so long she needs five precious minutes to get them into latex gloves. Sammy Rudovski is our driver, has been around a decade or two, and knows the drill. Generally he keeps quiet. Like all the ambulance drivers he is permitted to wear casual clothes, and on this festival night is decked out in a three-piece denim suit. None of them is happy about being on shift while the rest of the country is celebrating.

Like the sound of witches round a cauldron, regular cackles of laughter emanate from the front cabin. The witch analogy is not about evil spells, but rather the wicked sense of humour they share with ambulance workers worldwide.

Just over the river, in the shade of the ancient Kale Fort, we pull up and Dr Aquarius slides back the perspex peep window.

'Benja, we have a heart problems!' she shouts.

I appreciate her informing me, as the usual indication I get that we have been given a job is when the ambulance suddenly careens into oncoming traffic with the cry of a siren, throwing me off my seat. Riding in the back like a pet dog is not my idea of a good time. There are few windows and it's hot, stuffy and claustrophobic.

After a few minutes we move back and forth between apartment buildings; down the driveway of one, reversing up again, going around in circles. Most blocks are identical to one another and confusion is common. When we finally find the address Sammy has picked it by little more than a tiny number scrawled on a wall in white chalk.

Dr Aquarius leads the ascent up a graffiti-sprayed stairwell to the eighth floor carrying her little black doctor's bag containing a blood pressure cuff, stethoscope, her leopard-skin purse and cigarettes. When I see her do this I lament the many backbreaking years I have lugged every box and piece of equipment to top floor apartments without cause.

By the time we reach the fifth level with three to go, nurse Spazovska is gasping loudly behind me. Like a commando in the jungle, Dr Aquarius motions with her hand for us to stop. We pause a little for Spazovska to catch her breath, and she's no picture of health. Her heart and lungs are shot by years of relentless fagging, her arteries clogged with Macedonian cheese. Needless to say, performing this job on a regular basis in a city of apartment blocks without elevators ought to keep her in better shape.

By the time we reach the patient's door, Snezhana Spazovska seems close to respiratory arrest. Our patient, on the other hand, is calmly sipping a cup of tea. There must have been a mix-up, he says. He made it very clear to the call-taker that what he had done was slam his finger in a door. There's no question that slamming a finger in a door is painful, but calling an emergency doctor and nurse to apply an ice pack hardly seems reasonable.

It surprises me this one has slipped past the control room at Budapest Hospital. When I sat with them a week ago I'd become convinced that only the meanest nurses were assigned to work there. Every second emergency call received would have them abusing the caller for not being sick or injured enough to warrant an ambulance. Phones were continuously slammed down in the ears of helpless victims as services were refused outright.

Nurse Spazovska is pale and sweaty and can barely speak. She leans over the patient's glass coffee table while Dr Aquarius – who no doubt has seen this all before – rubs her back. Just for a moment I wonder whether I'm witnessing some drama created to give the man with his bruised finger a demonstration of what a *real* sick person looks like.

'I … my … is … tachycardia,' Spazovska splutters.

It's bad news when someone with shortness of breath speaks like this, catching air between each word.

Her heart is doing double-time when I take her pulse, convincing me she's genuine enough. Meanwhile the guy with the finger looks on with confusion. Despite our offers, Spazovska refuses medication and we patiently wait ten minutes for her to regain her composure. A recovery of sorts is made but it's no way to be starting a night shift.

Macedonia is a guarded nation with a great suspicion of outsiders and not many places have had me feeling more like a foreign agent than Skopje. No one gives much away here. Few people are open or candid. Faces are stony, scrutinising you with narrowed eyes. This is understandable considering the country's communist history, not to mention that 'a writer is something of a spy' as Graham Greene once wrote in *Stamboul Train*. Thanks to a shared block of Schogetten Stracciatella chocolate, the ambulance team now considers me a true colleague and that respect is unreserved.

Zoran Kostovski, the Australian Honorary Consul in Skopje, is a man with incredible personal energy and vibrant enthusiasm. He is also connected at every level of government thanks to the success of his private company, Motiva, which he started after reading *Body Language* by Australian author Allan Pease. The objective of Motiva is to provide its clients with training in superior communication techniques – particularly of the non-verbal variety – and it is through his delivery of these workshops to politicians that Zoran has not only befriended Nikola Gruevski, Macedonia's current prime minister but, to my great fortune, the current health minister, Dr Bujar Osmani.

When I first shared a bottle of Macedonian wine with Zoran he revealed there were only ever ten or fifteen Australians with no family connection to Macedonia visiting the country at any one time and that despite this minuscule number, they managed to keep him busy round the clock. This may have sounded like a complaint had Zoran not reassured me that he thoroughly enjoyed the entertainment his position afforded him. There was a poet who fell off his chair and fractured his hip. 'Dangerous work, poetry,' he said. Not long after, he was called to the police station for a female with schizophrenia found wandering the streets of Skopje in a state of undress. She had run out of medication while on holiday. Then there was the man who got so depressed after arriving in the drab city he promptly threw himself out of the second-storey window of his hotel. As anyone in ambulance work knows, the second storey is a half-arsed attempt at suicide. Once, I tell Zoran, I went to a man threatening to jump off the first level of a high-rise parking station. Ridiculous. Most interesting of all, says Zoran, was the man from Melbourne who arrived in Skopje at the time of the Victorian bushfires wearing little more than shorts and a T-shirt, carrying a handful of possessions in a small plastic bag. Apparently he wanted to get as far away from the fire as he could.

My request to meet the health minister, in order to acquire permission to join ambulance crews in Skopje, was a comparatively easy one, Zoran assures me. 'And he's an outstanding guy, in the toughest job, trying to do his best to bring reform.'

Indeed, on the day I'm meant to meet Dr Osmani, the front page of every newspaper shows hospital doctors walking off the job in protest at their low wages. In Macedonia, public hospital doctors earn little more than 400 euros a month, while nurses get 350 euros. Because the average rent is around 150 euros and electricity in the winter another 100 euros on top of that, most in the medical profession cannot even afford to visit a restaurant or have a drink in a bar. The wages are so low that over time it has become common practice to ask patients for money. Jumping the queue for surgery is achieved with cash alone and those without it may wait for a decade. The poor have enough trouble getting a prescription.

There is probably never a good time for an Australian paramedic to take tea with the health minister of a country burdened by such challenges. Nevertheless, I was invited to do so by Zoran and we sat in the very pleasant company of a softly spoken Osmani as he elaborated on his work.

Most significantly, his effort to stop kickbacks in the form of over-supplied medical materials to hospitals has put many of his public hospital doctors offside. At a Holiday Inn conference in 2008, Zoran introduced Dr Osmani to a patient classification software developed by Australia that keeps track of hospital resources and is known as the Australian Refined Diagnosis Related Groups (AR-DRG) system. Many countries suffering the effects of health service corruption have installed this program with enormous success, including Saudi Arabia, Greece and Romania. On behalf of the prime minister, Zoran negotiated the purchase of the AR-DRG software by Macedonia for a very modest price. Two years later it is 'still in the process' of being installed. Across Macedonia, hospital heads have made every effort to block its introduction, revealing just how many people are dependent on medical supplies kickbacks to supplement their incomes. As effective as the AR-DRG system may be, it does not address this root cause of corruption.

As for my placement on ambulances of Skopje, Dr Osmani has no objection and simply warns me not to injure myself. He is unconcerned I might pen something critical about the Macedonian health system. 'It wouldn't be news,' he says. 'Everyone knows the country is poor. Why should we pretend it to be otherwise?'

At a roadside kiosk Dr Aquarius buys us bottles of Pimp Juice, a local soft drink we sip through straws on the way to the next job. Earlier in the week I saw a billboard for the beverage depicting a smiling gangster with gold teeth. This is what many of the young men look like in Shutka, the capital of gypsies, and I wonder if it's bottled there.

For my benefit Sammy takes the ambulance past the house of Esma Redzepova, known globally as the Gypsy Queen, a singer whose remarkable voice carries the collective emotions of the Roma, and whose music I have followed for some time. In opposition to those who react angrily to being labelled a gypsy, Redzepova encourages the Roma to be proud of the term and has always used the earnings from her record sales to distribute free medicine to the poor.

A little further on, near Topaana, one of the earliest gypsy *maalos,* stands the ominous new American embassy. Rumour has it this is not just *any* embassy. The complex is so vast one would need an hour to walk around it. Much to the dismay of Topaana gypsies it has also taken up every inch of what was once the beloved city park they used for weddings and picnics, forcing them onto a small, cramped traffic island in the embassy's shadow.

Just off the Krimska Road, a family of rotund Macedonians has had a fierce argument during which the father has shattered a framed photograph of his wife and stormed from the house leaving her and his three adult children in a state of hysteria. The two daughters, both in their mid-thirties, are howling uncontrollably on the lounge while a younger man, probably in his late twenties, kneels at his mother's feet sobbing. One would think the woman's husband had passed away, but he has only gone to the pub. Were it not for the fact we attend jobs like this every day in Skopje I would not be so cynical. Nor would I be wondering why so many simple disagreements in this country result in group hyperventilation or all-out brawls.

Dr Aquarius tries to calm the lady, gives it about a minute or so, looks at her watch, then twitches an over-plucked eyebrow at nurse Spazovska and rolls up the sleeves of her lab coat. Spazovska knows the drill and opens a black briefcase she has taken into the house. In it are rows of glittering glass ampoules tinkling like little wind chimes whenever she handles them. It's pretty much all the nurses ever carry, the drugs – the first line of emergency care in Macedonia. The only other items apart from medications are cotton balls for swabbing, needles and saline, and a bunch of thin candles to light for the dead. With nimble fingers Spazovska removes an ampoule of Valium 10 milligrams, snaps its neck, draws it up and hands it to Dr Aquarius.

Seconds after stabbing it in, without further ado, we are out the door.

Valium, valium, valium. Half the briefcase is full of the stuff. At a guess there'd be at least twenty ampoules in there and even that is not enough some nights. Morphine supplies may be out of stock, while some doctors buy aspirin for heart patients with their own money. But the Valium never dries up. This surprises me as the drug is dispensed like candy. So popular is Valium in this city that it is common for ambulance crews to administer 'one for the patient and one for the relative'. Balkan funerals are the worst. At these there can be fifty, even a hundred, distressed mourners demanding a shot.

Our next job – or 'invitation' as the medics endearingly call them – is to a woman with high blood pressure and a headache. Again, along with a prescription for Monopril and a beta-blocker comes intramuscular Valium.

'We take the Pimp Juice, they take the Valium,' laughs Dr Aquarius afterwards. 'That is how the world goes round!'

An hour later everyone is thrilled to have discovered an apartment block with an elevator, none happier than our smoking asthmatic nurse. On the top floor a man has been vomiting for a week. Exciting stuff, I think to myself.

The apartment is painted a deep red and decorated with kitsch throne-like furniture more suited to a medieval castle than a tiny bachelor pad. Gold candelabras rest on a narrow black table in the centre of the room along with a giant porcelain tiger and a vase of plastic irises. Macedonians have less money now than they did in the communist era yet give the impression they are enjoying the spoils of capitalism. All over former Yugoslavia one can find this same quasi-bourgeois aesthetic. If you want to know how a two-dollar shop can make you look rich, just ask a Macedonian.

When Snezhana Spazovska removes a hideous oil painting of a teary-eyed clown from above the lounge where our patient is lying I am momentarily relieved. Unfortunately she has not taken it down to improve the appearance of the man's apartment but to hang an IV drip on the hook in its place.

The moment she has done this, we leave.

Not one of the three jobs we have knocked over before sundown has had us on scene for more than five minutes and not one patient has been transported to hospital. Only yesterday, a Skopje steelworks employee with a bleeding nose, a case I would normally spend ten minutes or so treating with manual pressure alone, was handled completely differently. Pharmacology was the mainstay and the patient was fixed in half the time. There were jabs of Valium and Frusemide and a cotton ball soaked in adrenalin shoved up the nostril. Again less than five minutes on scene and no transport. Although it could be argued that a certain thoroughness and continuum of care may be lacking here, the Franco-German model of pre-hospital intervention is so far proving highly efficient. In most other countries where I've worked, all these patients would by now be clogging up emergency departments. As for the man with vomiting and dehydration lying there on his over-ornate lounge with a drip in his arm, what happens when the solution has run through?

'We give instruction on how to remove it,' says Spazovska, 'How to stop his vein from bleeding. We explain him procedure, don't worry.'

To a paramedic from a system without physicians such a practice seems daring. Not every patient is bright enough or possessed of the nerves to remove their own cannula and stem a bleed. But these, it seems, are considered worthwhile risks to save a tenuous hospital system from being overburdened.

Our assigned station for the night lies in the somewhat forlorn suburb of Chaiar, not far from Shutka. After a couple of home visits in the Albanian quarter issuing Tramadol to cancer patients, our driver, Sammy, passes the house of Johann the Killer, the commander of a police unit responsible for war crimes against an Albanian village and currently awaiting trial in The Hague. It's a purple and mauve monstrosity hung with wagon wheels and cowboy paraphernalia, complete with a ten-foot medieval gate. Sammy is also Albanian and finds it incredible the house remains untouched. As we head to Chaiar he tells me how last month a patient refused to get into an ambulance driven by an Albanian and subsequently threatened the crew with a steak knife.

Ethnic tensions run deep in Macedonia. My friends here, even the young and university educated, frequently shock me with their overt racism towards Albanian Muslims. No one even bothers beginning with the customary 'I'm not racist, but ...' preface as racists in Australia often do. Perhaps this tension is understandable when the last skirmish of gunfire exchanged between Macedonian forces and Albanian insurgents occurred as recently as 2001. And it is only since 2007 that Macedonians dare to walk through the Old City dominated by mosques and ancient bath-houses separated by the worn cobble streets winding to a Turkish bazaar.

Then there is the issue of Vodno, the steep mountain high above Skopje where Macedonians have installed the Millennium Cross, the largest crucifix in the world, sixty-six metres tall. Without a hint of shame my friends admit the cross was placed as a mark of territory rather than a symbol of Christ's grace and tolerance; ethnic Albanians should be constantly reminded who the rightful owners of the city are. Even by night, from the window of the ambulance when everything is black, the cross on Vodno hovers, brightly lit and imposing against the night sky. It may be a thing of beauty but for me it's a beauty tainted by the country's godless divisiveness.

At Chaiar Station, a sweet Albanian nurse with near-perfect English is manning the radio and scissoring small squares of gauze from a giant sheet for sterilisation. Her name is Drenusha Arneri and in our earlier conversations she admitted it took her a year to feel accepted by her colleagues. Now, despite being a Muslim, she celebrates Easter with them, helps colour eggs at the ambulance station and even brings along a plate of homemade baklava. Under Dr Maja Poposka the service has come a long way in creating a positive environment. Whenever she can spare one, Poposka even sends an ambulance to Mecca with a team of Albanian medics onboard to help out.

For Dr Maja Poposka nature helps her deal with stress and that is why in the middle of her office at Bucharest Hospital she keeps a giant indoor tree growing in a pot with branches reaching out around the room and leaning like a friend across her desk. By all appearances this chain-smoking doctor is more Russian supermodel than ambulance service director. Before taking up her position two years ago she had already worked fifteen years on ambulances in Skopje, roughly the same time I have worked on them in Australia.

'Everything I have seen,' she says matter-of-factly.

We begin a discussion on the improvements made to Macedonia's ambulances since she became director. New ambulances donated from around Europe, white uniforms for the medical staff, better training and equipment. It is hard to believe, but up until 2006 none of Skopje's ambulances had defibrillators on board. Response times were notoriously dismal and the ambulance doctors had a countrywide reputation for being mean and rude.

To some extent, from my random canvassing of locals I have met here, public perception of Skopje 194 is still rather poor. At a taxi stand in town not a single driver could recite the emergency number and an informal survey I conducted at a Bob Marley tribute party in a city park revealed the widespread opinion that ambulances still take forever to arrive and are staffed by 'bitches' anyway. Neither of these perceptions is at all fair, as I've discovered first hand, and I ask Dr Poposka why the service has not done a better job of public relations since she took office.

'Problem is we cannot advertise our improvements,' she replies. 'It is better for us to go about our work quietly and rely on word of mouth. You see, we are still under-resourced and only just manage to meet the eight minutes response time standard for 90 per cent of top priority cases. What will happen if we tell the world how good we are now, how quick and polite and professional we have become?'

It's true that public ambulance services do not generally benefit from advertising. The better a service looks the more people will call, leading to a higher demand that will negatively impact on response times. The only publicity campaigns an ambulance service should probably entertain are those that concern prevention and discourage calling for inappropriate reasons. This is a vastly more difficult campaign for a service with general practitioners on every ambulance and a public that knows it.

Maja Poposka's frustrations working on the road prompted her to apply for the top job when the former boss retired. Four old Russian-built Lada station wagons are still parked in the basement of the ambulance headquarters, cobwebbed and rusty. Only a few years ago they were all the city had.

'You can imagine our reputation, driving around Skopje in these things,' said Dr Poposka when she took me to see them. 'We were always late and even then we couldn't do much for the really sick ones. See, look how low the roof is. None of us ever did CPR in these cars, impossible.'

'So what did you do in cardiac arrests?'

'Drive fast.'

Hearing this I understand completely her reasons for leading the service. Watching people die from a lack of space would be maddening for any ambulance worker, let alone a medical doctor.

Behind her office lies a larger ambulance graveyard containing numerous donated vehicles from around Europe, all hand-me-downs still bearing the logos of their former masters. Here I saw a Johanniter Mercedes from the Germans, a 118 van from Rome and a French Renault from the SAMU. Up until recently Skopje 194 used these vehicles as they were. On any one day it was common to see ambulances from various European nations all screaming through Skopje at the same time. This reminded me of a friend who had visited Fiji and happened upon the same ambulance he had driven around Sydney for years being used there since its donation to the country a year earlier.

Chaiar Station is little more than a few cold rooms in the wing of a small clinic, lit by a tiny television with bad reception that everyone put in for. Few want to miss the Macedonian version of *Wheel of Fortune* known here as *Wheel of Happiness*. For those who know that money does not guarantee happiness, the game show is followed by an addictive Turkish soap opera. As we settle in to watch the next episode of *Yabanci Damat*, Drenousha helps us get into the spirit of things by serving Turkish coffee.

Ambulance stations of Macedonia become drop-in medical centres after hours and on the weekends. So an additional doctor is always on duty at night and has a separate consultation room. For the festival night of Saint Nicholas, Dr Save Bobonovski is on shift, his first name ensuring great popularity among his patients. At one time he also worked on the ambulances, but that was ten years ago and he quit after attending a nasty accident at Alexander the Great Airport. On 5 March 1993, eighty-three people died when flight crew forgot to de-ice a Macedonian Airlines Fokker prior to departure and it crashed seconds after take-off. Save was first on the scene. As he tells it, bodies and body parts were scattered as far as the eye could see. He decided soon after he was more suited to working indoors.

A second crew comes by on their way to a chest pain and picks up an ECG machine. At present there are not enough to go round and Chaiar ambulances have to share a single ancient Hellige box with its little rubber suckers and wide leather straps that bind to wrists and ankles and around the chest. It must hark from the 1960s or thereabouts and looks more KGB than ECG. We've used it plenty of times, and vintage though the Hellige may be, it is still a functional 12-lead cardiograph.

Dr Aquarius scoffs. 'Our government doesn't have money for new ECG machines, but they sure have it for bronze lions in public squares. Have you ever seen a bronze lion save a life?'

To boost morale, reinvigorate patriotism and attract tourists, the government of Macedonia has created a controversial building project known as Skopje 2014. By crossing the old stone bridge over the Vardar River in the direction of the central mosque, one can see where work on the multimillion denar project has begun. A highly fanciful preview of what the completed dream may look like is also available on YouTube as a musical montage. Ridiculous oversized monuments are superimposed on city intersections, including a sky-scraping Alexander atop his rearing horse in the main square. Imitation baroque buildings line the banks of the Vardar where a troupe of dancing fountains shoot from the murky rapids.

Continued Greek denial of Macedonian identity is certainly part of what has prompted Skopje 2014. But for unemployed and hungry Macedonians it is all too much.

'Remember how Ceausescu died in Romania?' says Dr Aquarius. 'He built an *Arc de Triomphe* replica in Bucharest while his people were starving and was executed by firing squad.'

There is a patient with shortness of breath in Shutka, where we spend most of our time each shift. As in the films of Emir Kusturica and their endless parties of drunken gypsies firing pistols into the air, breaking bottles over each other's heads and tripping over roaming geese, the *maalo* has an atmosphere of madness even in the absence of wedding receptions. Still, we are rarely called to trauma cases. There is surprisingly little violence in Shutka considering the quantity of the homebrew, *rakija*, the inhabitants consume. They are not a violent race. Never have the gypsies fought a war or occupied a land.

In contrast to the guarded personalities of many Macedonians, the gypsies are warmer and quicker to smile. Perhaps they feel secure and at peace here. Macedonia may be over-spending public money on bronze lions and flaming crucifixes, but the country has arguably the most compassionate policy towards the Roma anywhere in Europe. By comparison, Italy and France spent much of 2010 gypsy hunting. Although they weren't shot, as happened under the Nazis in World War II, gypsies were rounded up like cattle and forced back to Romania and Bulgaria. Many were not from these countries in the first place. It's hard to know what land, if any, a gypsy calls home. Since migrating from India a thousand years ago, they have spread to all corners of the earth and are regularly uprooted and chased away by governments.

Macedonia, however, has allowed gypsies the right to identify as Roma, to live in their own suburb and to have a representative in parliament. With its own mayor, permanent housing and radio stations, it is no wonder Shutka has become host to the largest number of gypsies anywhere.

Not everyone in Shutka is satisfied. Many are disappointed the government is not doing more to help them. Social security is only available to those Roma registered as residents of Macedonia and even then it is a paltry 50 euros a month. With some notable exceptions, including a handful of doctors and lawyers, the Roma are not much interested in education and few end up qualified for decent work. This forces many to rely on the garbage collection, the begging and the thievery for which they are known. Attending a school or a job to become a cog in society holds little appeal. More thrilling are horses and music and fire, all things wild and free, living each day as if it were the last.

Finding an address in Shutka can take a while. Some of the streets are cracked and deeply gouged with potholes and the eccentric little homes rendered in lurid colours have all kinds of madcap decorations hanging on their outside walls, from obscure coats-of-arms to enormous cuckoo clocks. But street numbers on letterboxes are scarce. We stop and ask a group of men sharing a foot-long salami and *rakija* if they know where our patient lives. After some lengthy argument they point toward the bazaar. Sometimes, even in serious emergencies, we drive around the *maalo* in dizzy confusion, following several opposing directions.

Thankfully, the streets are easy to remember. Without a shred of irony the Roma have given them names like Washington Square Boulevard, John F Kennedy Parade and Disneyland. Shoddily constructed miniature palaces of concrete can be found here. Poorer homes, in many cases, shanty-style shacks are more likely found along Che Guevara Drive, Shakespeare Avenue and Garcia Lorca Lane. At the bottom of the hill there is a quarter of Shutka I have visited that looks no different to a Bombay slum, complete with muddy passages, huts constructed from junk and United Nations water pumps.

Past the smugglers' bazaar where toothless old men sell lacy bras hanging in rows along rusty fences, where bootleg perfumes and pointless porcelain pigs go for a steal, we pull up at a partially collapsed building and enter a 2-metre-square room, home to a family of seven. Our patient is a forty-year-old woman with six children and a husband in jail. Only a gypsy can peel potatoes while suffering severe respiratory distress, I think to myself. Her mouth is snapping with every breath, as if biting for air.

Everyone seems to have breathing problems in Shutka. It's either asthma or emphysema or bronchitis or all of these at once. Temperatures in winter can drop to minus 20 degrees. If there is rain the streets of Shutka become rivers of freezing mud and many of the children do not have boots. Chest infections are common. Adults sit all day and night in crowded rooms, chain-smoking the contraband Marlboro their children passively inhale.

Dr Aquarius and Snezhana Spazovska don't mess about. They promptly administer an injection of Amyphyline and Dexamethasone during which the woman only momentarily ceases her potato peeling. It surprises me that oxygen is rarely given to patients the crew intends on leaving at home, especially those with breathing problems. On this occasion Dr Aquarius is feeling generous and runs the patient on a low rate through nasal prongs for several minutes, though staying on scene too long in the *maalo* is unwise. News of an ambulance entering the ghetto quickly gets around and it's only a matter of time – often less than fifteen minutes – before every sick person with the slightest complaint surfaces for treatment. Suddenly the ambulance becomes a mobile clinic and is trapped indefinitely. Many gypsies are not registered citizens and have no entitlement to hospital treatment. For them, the only hope of getting medical help is to bail up ambulances whenever they see them and appeal to the compassion of the doctor on board to get a free consultation.

The sun has dropped below the snow-capped Shari Mountain Range when we pull up at a small house so crooked it could have been built by a child. It is dark as a cave inside and the floor is covered in the shapes of countless bodies wetly snoring under thick floral blankets. A woman who does not bother brushing the hair from her face rolls over and pulls down an edge of her grimy tracksuit pants, exposing a buttock.

Dr Aquarius sighs and nods at nurse Spazovska who flicks open her black briefcase again, cracks a few ampoules, draws them up and stabs them in. The woman pulls the blanket over her head, falls back to sleep and we are out the door.

Two minutes and thirty-five seconds and not a word exchanged between medic and patient.

'Did you know her?' I ask, perplexed.

'Not personally,' says Dr Aquarius, climbing back into the ambulance.

'How did you guess what was wrong with her? Or what to give her?'

'You should understand by now. When they want an injection straight up it's the same thing every time. Vitamin B1, B6, B12 and C for good measure.'

If they're agitated, Valium is part of the cocktail too. And gypsies are notoriously prone to agitation. Should the Valium run out, the doctor will resort to aqua injections – plain water or normal saline. Few patients know any better. It is not about the drug anyway but about the *spritz*. With the exception of heroin addicts I've never met a patient enthusiastic about injections. Many Roma, however, can't get enough. This is because they have what Dr Aquarius calls 'injection jealousy'. Should a gypsy observe her neighbour receiving two vitamin injections from an ambulance crew, she will later call up and try to outdo her rival by asking for three. Roma are very jealous people. Angry scenes occur if ambulance crews don't give the maximum number of injections, regardless of whether the patient needs them or not.

'Once, in Shutka alone, I gave one hundred and thirty injections over a single week,' boasts Snezhana Spazovska through the slide window.

Seems to me a bad precedent has been set. A community expectation has been established from which these medics find it difficult to escape.

'Most of the time the Rom are very peaceful,' says Dr Aquarius. 'But, well, we give as many injections of Valium or vitamins or aqua as it takes us to get out of there quickly. It is not only Rom. Other Macedonians are like this too. No patient in our country is satisfied without a *spritz*.'

Injections are a matter of service efficiency rather than pandering. If a crew decides to leave without giving a jab, the patient is likely to wait fifteen minutes or so then call again. Indeed, they will call and call until they get an ambulance crew willing to give them one. Repeat callers are not unique to Macedonia and are a problem anywhere, in any country. Some callers in Australia are known to have our easy-to-remember three-digit emergency number on speed dial. In exasperation, some paramedics manage this problem by transporting the patient to hospital to remove them from their home phones so they won't call again. Of course, this simply shifts the problem. Treating patients in the field is more desirable, but whether it is ethical to inject a patient for the sake of operational efficiency alone is an interesting question. Maybe a little bending of the rules is justified for the greater good, allowing ambulances to be more readily available for life-threatening cases. I can't help thinking, however, that if injection-jealous gypsies knew that the party was over, the call volume would drop and the burden would ease naturally.

Girls with gold hoop earrings smile and wave and kick up bright floral dresses as we pass them trailing a mob of grubby children. Their look is a welcome flashback to the gypsy aesthetic of old in a township where most of the women have long ago discovered Adidas and cheap bling.

We pull up outside a peppermint-green house with a waterfall feature built against the front wall. Inside a middle-aged woman lies theatrically collapsed on the hallway carpet, hyperventilating. A dozen family members and relatives shuffle in behind us to have a look.

Dr Aquarius asks the woman a few questions, which she answers with excessive gasping and groaning and rolling about. Spazovska is next to me and whispers, 'Pain all over.'

Right. Pain all over. As if I couldn't have picked it, that classic ailment of the chronic neurotic. How it makes us laugh when we hear it! Not in front of the patient – *never* in front of the patient. Oh, but how we laugh. From what I can tell, Dr Aquarius is examining the patient in the same manner I do in such cases. Slowly she palpates every region of the woman's body. What about here? And what about here? And here? And every time the woman groans or winces or pulls away, even when Dr Aquarius has reached and squeezed the tip of her pinky finger. What drives an unusually thorough examination like this is a hope that our looks of confusion in response to the patient's unspecific complaints will be a hint to her and her relatives that we are not convinced and that perhaps, to avoid embarrassment, someone should put an end to the entertainment before we are forced to do so in the back of the ambulance.

'She requesting something special,' Spazovska says.

Gypsies love a bit of drama. This I can appreciate – life is great when it's thrilling. Less forgivable are the patients who have an ambulance called for the sake of attracting attention. Attention-seeking exists in every country and in every cultural group, and is particularly prevalent in very large families. A person feeling left out or snubbed for some reason may decide that by feigning a medical emergency they will get what they crave. The strategy usually works well and they soon find their extended family standing around them saying pointless things like, 'Oh my God! Oh my God! Oh my God!' and rushing wet towels from the bathroom. Perfect! So long as their symptoms are as ambiguous as 'pain all over' and appear severe enough, the little fakers may even get a ride to hospital. Of course, on arrival they will make a miraculous recovery and discharge themselves before a doctor has even seen them.

Because these are delicate situations I wait out the front of the house. From where I stand I can see a ten-metre cherry tree belonging to a regular emphysema patient. A week ago I was up that tree picking cherries for her as she'd complained about being too old and breathless to climb a ladder. After that day Kass and I ate cherries for breakfast, lunch and dinner.

The adult daughter of the drama queen comes out and forces a cigarette between my lips. Her smile reveals a big gold tooth flashing in the sun. She wears yellow lycra leggings and a decorative red belt with a playboy bunny buckle. After she lights my cigarette she puts her hand on my shoulder and comes very near.

'You are married?' she asks directly.

I nod.

'Not matter for me,' she purrs, exhaling smoke in my face.

With a daughter like this it's no wonder the patient has pain all over, I think. What kind of woman tries seducing the medic while her mother is near death?

From inside the house comes the sound of yelling. Something crashes and breaks. This is followed by a short scream after which Dr Aquarius saunters out, peels off her gloves and gives a wink.

'She not wishes to come with us,' says the doctor.

Sometimes it seems the crew is more effective when their international guest is not in the room.

Intense verbal exchanges are the norm in Macedonia. What sounds like an argument may be just as likely the whispering of lovers elsewhere. Macedonians, like Italians, Greeks and Arabs, for that matter, can have a simple interaction about the weather while sounding like they're about to strangle each other.

An exchange like this occurred during one of my many meetings with ambulance service director Maja Poposka. The afternoon started badly when she showed me a video clip of a major incident exercise on a highway near the Serbian border. The footage had been set to a heart-wrenching song, *Game Without Limits* by Tose Proeski, a young Macedonian singer recently killed in a car accident. His death had been traumatic for the entire country.

'I chose this song because I like it very much,' Poposka tells me, looking off into the middle distance, just holding back her tears. 'Sometimes in our profession we also push the limits.'

There is so much she could have meant by this, but I sensed she was referring to the risks, both physical and mental, that ambulance workers subject themselves to. Surrounded by craziness, by things going wrong, by lives twisted up, we risk losing perspective on our own reality. If this happens, anything is possible in terms of our personal behaviour. If we lose our grasp on rational thought our work may indeed become a game without limits.

We talked then at length about adrenalin and its toll on us

over time, finding common ground in our mutual experience of adrenalin withdrawal. My wife Kass has often wondered how it's possible for me to be so upbeat at work, even at the end of a rough day, yet arrive home grumpy. When adrenalin wears off some of us simply 'crash'. Adrenalin is, after all, a type of high. It creates euphoria and for this reason people engage in all manner of dangerous activities to pursue it. But like every other high, it is only *high* because it is preceded and followed by a *low* and ambulance workers are by no means immune. Indeed, some even orchestrate drama in their private lives to maintain their adrenalin levels artificially.

It was about this time in the meeting that Boban Vivovski, the humpty-dumpty fleet manager, entered the room and said something to Poposka that didn't please her at all. A shouting match ensued. She slammed down her diary with an almighty slap, pushed her swivel chair out and chased Vivovski into the corridor. The door slammed shut behind her. Outside the room the argument continued, punctuated every now and then by a loud thud, as if one or both of them were whacking the wall or throwing the other against it. All I could do was remain in the shade of her indoor tree, quietly embarrassed, listening to them blowing up outside. For the CEO and her fleet manager to behave this naturally in front of me was surely an honour, though I would have been less concerned were it not the day after a Macedonian doctor at one of Skopje's main hospitals stabbed her fellow doctor seventeen times in a fit of rage. On the television they said she had a 'brain snap'. As the scene of this stabbing played out in my mind while listening to the yelling in the corridor, I swallowed hard.

When Dr Poposka came back into the room, unscathed, she sat down and let out a sigh, giving me a measured smile.

'It's not only the gypsies who are passionate peoples. Anyway, I would rather yell at my fleet manager than at my road staff. You will never hear me yell at ambulance teams. They work hard and don't deserve it. They are my friends and I always take a cigarette with them. Without their respect I can achieve nothing.'

One day, when Dr Poposka is tired of her position, she would consider working the road again and wants to be sure her legacy as director will not make her unwelcome there. As for the conflict among her management team, she insists it is 'a type of love'. In my opinion she is suffering from plain and simple adrenalin withdrawal. For a former ambulance doctor there is a clear excitement deficit that comes with a management position and the office environment. Yelling matches and fist-fights are, one could say, the methadone of adrenalin withdrawal.

Evidence of the Roma's Indian origins can be seen on walls we pass in the ambulance, white painted designs identical to those I have come across in small desert villages of Rajasthan and Gujarat.

We follow two boys running towards the Shutka bazaar clutching trumpets. Their eyes in our headlights are wide with excitement. The smell of barbecuing lamb wafts through the open windows of our ambulance and in the distance we can hear the sound of a brass band playing. When we reach the intersection of the bazaar a large crowd of gypsies surrounds a group of men on horns and drums. Slowly we edge the ambulance through a throng of scruffy kids with bleached spiky hair and gold chains dancing wildly. Their look is hip-hop but their moves are pure fireside Bollywood.

'This will be us at 3 am,' laughs Dr Aquarius. Snezhana Spazovska giggles and Sammy yelps the siren and waves at the mob. Some of the kids whistle in return and drum their hands on the ambulance as we go by.

'We are now going to village in the hills,' says Dr Aquarius. 'The sun is down. You know what it means when sun is down on festival of Saint Nicholas?'

'Gets dark?'

'Time to party.'

As if on cue Sammy cranks the stereo and frantic turbo-folk music reverberates through the ambulance, thumping like a gangster car. When he steps on the accelerator the G-forces pitch me back into the treatment seat. Along ripped-up mountain roads we go at ridiculous speeds. Without available restraints it's not long before I'm as battered as a turnip on a truck. They must have got a call to a car accident or heart attack victim or something equally serious as Sammy takes every craterous pothole dead-on, bouncing me so high my head slams into the ceiling.

Ten minutes later we park by a grand house precariously perched on a hillside. Sammy comes round and pulls open the side door. I stagger out, my body predicting bruises in the morning.

'Now we eat,' he smiles. 'Come.'

We are welcomed by Igor – an ambulance colleague on his night off – who leads us into a dining room where a long table is ringed by a dozen people and spread from one end to the other with platters of food: savoury pastries, smoked pork, cheeses, salads and *sarma* rolls.

'Sit! Sit! Sit! Welcome! Sit!' commands our jolly host as the other guests shuffle around to let the ambulance crew in. 'Eat! Eat! Eat!'

We're all quite hungry and don't need a second invitation.

'Don't eat too much,' advises Dr Aquarius with a wink. 'This is only our first stop, understanding?'

For the summer festival of Saint Nicholas it is customary for Macedonian families to prepare an ongoing banquet that lasts all night. Friends and family move freely from house to house, village to village, dropping in at will wherever they please, to eat and drink what is there before heading to the next home. Never is there an obligation to stay for longer than it takes to knock back a glass of *rakija*.

Igor puts a strong hand on my shoulder, bangs a small glass

down in front of me and fills it from a bottle of crystal-clear *rakija* inside of which is a miniature wooden ladder, as if inviting me to climb in.

'Drink! Drink! Drink!' Igor shouts at me.

Everyone is looking my way, at the foreign guest about to taste their *rakija*. It is customary in the Balkans to sample a family's home brew after entering a house and, if one values one's life, declaring it the best brandy one has ever tasted. Any reservations I have about drinking on shift are subdued by the fact that Sammy and nurse Snezhana Spazovska also have a fully laden glass of *rakija* in their hands, while Dr Aquarius is savouring a mixture of red wine and Coca-Cola known as *bamboos*. Unlike them, I am not treating patients or driving an ambulance or representing anyone in particular. In that case, what is the harm in it?

None at all, and down it goes.

It's a plum *rakija*, as the Macedonians prefer it, and it delivers a vicious punch to the guts after setting fire to the oesophagus. In saying that, it is not turpentine and has a subtle but detectable underlying flavour of stone fruit, and if the *rakija* contains high quantities of honey it's even more enjoyable. Either way, the liquor delivers both pleasure and pain, and is the beverage of choice for Macedonians and gypsies alike.

'Is good? Uncle Igor's *rakija* is good?'

'Is good, is good,' I reply.

The party breaks into approving applause, glasses clink and someone pulls out an accordion and begins to play. Everyone is in fine spirits.

We have been at Igor's for fifteen minutes when Dr Aquarius – now finishing off her second glass of *bamboos* – says we should keep rolling. This is not so we can return to our area for work but instead to visit the next home for another round of everything we have just ingested. We get up, offer our thanks and leave.

Once more we hurtle down perilous mountain roads and I'm

relieved when we reach the flatter pastures outside Skopje. Here we pull up at a farmhouse belonging to Yovan, an ambulance driver on his night off. As we climb through the arch in a hedge made dark by a cloud obscuring the moon I get an unexpected pang of joy and know right away the *rakija* has begun to speak.

Up a flight of stairs we go and into another room heavy with trapped cigarette smoke hovering over a banquet table set with baskets of bread and cold chicken. As expected, Yovan pours me a glass of his own *rakija*.

I hold up my hand in protest.

'Unprofessional,' I stutter helplessly.

Dr Aquarius looks over disapprovingly.

'Ah, Benja! What kind of stupid guest you are? Drink it up!'

And because she is a doctor, I do.

Nurse Spazovska crosses her legs and sips a glass of *ouzo* like a cocktail. Perhaps I will do the same with my *rakija*. Dr Aquarius is back on her *bamboos* and with a Marlboro in her other hand is as far removed as a doctor can get from being a health department pin-up. Yovan's wife heaps my plate with pita and marinated peppers, staring me down until I finish. While trying to read the body language of a lively conversation, I notice something odd about my glass of *rakija*. No matter how much I sip, it never gets any emptier. It's magic, bottomless. After fifteen minutes, when I'm beginning to feel rather giddy, I realise Yovan has been secretly topping it up whenever I turn away. By the time I cotton on to him and lodge my protest, the whole room is laughing.

'Benja, have you seen our city's most famous singer?' asks Dr Aquarius with a mischievous twinkle in her eye.

'Esma Redzepova?'

'No, not Esma. No, I mean, *Macedonian* singer. Her name is Double Double X Irena.'

Everyone giggles and Yovan is most pleased to hear the name.

'Oh, yes, yes, yes!' he says, clapping his hands.

With a name like that I wonder aloud if she sings with her clothes on.

'Well, yes,' says Dr Aquarius, ashing her cigarette. 'At first, but by the end of song there is less clothing than at the beginning, if you know what I mean.'

It's not the first time the doctor has brought up a risqué topic in our time together and I've begun to feel like an innocent boy rapidly corrupted. The night is thick with expectation and I get the feeling that anything could happen at any time. It's a tension paramedics thrive on, the unending surprises of our job, our ghost train, our comedy of horrors.

Interrupting the party is the sudden ringing of the emergency phone carried by Dr Aquarius in her lab coat.

'Everybody shhhhh!' she says, lifting her hand.

She takes the call and there is a hush that is normally impossible to achieve in a room full of tipsy Macedonians. But all of us sit patiently in silence. Yovan puffs quietly on a giant cigar, two of his kids mouth rude words to one another while a plate of rolled cabbage is passed around.

'Da ... da ... da,' says Dr Aquarius into the phone.

If only the crotchety controllers could see us now, miles from where they think we are, having a great time.

When the doctor hangs up everyone exhales in relief.

'Job in next village,' she says. 'It's not far, we have time to drink up.'

At this stage I'm unsure of whether or not I will be able to stand up, let alone drink up. Yes, I've always been a bit of a lightweight, but this is a whole new experience.

For a man with an uncountable number of brandy shots onboard, Sammy confidently clatters over an unpaved road to the next village without mishap. A trumpeting big band beats through my head and my body feels like it's going over Niagara Falls in a barrel. I'm beginning to see things too. 'Rakijallucinations' they call them. Bright sparkles of light encircling me like a wreath of fireworks. Kaleidoscopic fractals break up my peripheral vision and I enter a spiralling vortex of burning stars whenever I shut my eyes. A Balkan *rakija* is the sister of that devil's advocate, tequila.

I use the doorframe to prop myself up and observe Snezhana Spazovska and Dr Aquarius treating an elderly lady with dehydration. I cannot understand it. The two medics seem dead straight. Better still, they are far friendlier to the patient than I've ever seen them be before. As they set up a drip I go outside and Sammy turns the ambulance headlights off so I can take a swaying pee against a tractor. I marvel at its giant tyres. Then I gaze out over a moonlit radish field behind the farmhouse, overcome by its chrome-like beauty.

When Dr Aquarius climbs back into the front seat of the ambulance I ask her how it is possible to set up a drip after so many *bamboos*.

'Benja! We are Macedonians! After three bottles of *ouzo* I never miss a vein! Tell me, are veins sober? No! They are dancing around and falling over and disappearing and reappearing and are too much cheeky!'

So it takes a tipsy medic to understand a tipsy vein. What, with the good morale, a cheerful approach to patients and apparently better clinical performance, I'm surprised a regular nip of *rakija* is not service policy.

Smoke wafts from the dividing window when Nurse Spazovska slides it back and says, 'We go Shutka now for gypsy magic!'

I groan my acknowledgement.

No longer able to hold myself in the treatment seat and feeling rather queasy I roll onto the stretcher and grasp hold of the side rails as Sammy drives like a rollercoaster. The stretcher rattles under me until I recall that it's broken and doesn't lock in. For weeks my job on the ambulance has been to hold it in place so patients don't fly out the back. *The Disorderly Orderly* comes to mind, an old film where comedian Jerry Lewis careers for fifteen minutes down urban streets on a runaway ambulance trolley. Still, I'm too sick to get off. Everything in the ambulance sounds like it's about to dislodge. I hear the jittering of every pair of tweezers and scissors, every safety pin, every latch and buckle and cable, everything shaking and squeaking; a cacophony so deafening I'm convinced the whole patient compartment is ready to come off its fixture and catapult through the cabbage fields.

Rarely, if ever, does a paramedic have the misfortune of riding as a patient, flat on their back and backwards to an uncertain destination. But that is how I find myself, crippled by Macedonian liquor, watching the glowing streetlights through the window as they flash by in hypnotic succession.

Deep in the Shutka *maalo* a chronically ill gypsy woman we visited a week ago has passed away. New Life Avenue – the aptly named street where her house stands – is thronged with relatives while neighbours swarm around our ambulance. Inside, the old lady is laid out, her complexion waxy-white, her mouth open wide. Two dozen people sit around the room looking forlorn, passing a flask of *rakija* between them.

Out in the courtyard is the dead woman's sister, her face of hard years framed by a brightly spangled shawl. Her hoop earrings glint in the light of an overhead bulb. When she sees us she begins to sing an ancient song in a rasping, heart-wrenching voice. Everyone listens intently. Everything is surreal. Quiet grief pours out of each person here. So moving is the sister's song, my heart is hurting for the woman I never knew. On a card table nearby, tears belonging to Dr Aquarius fall onto the death certificate. She tries her best to dab it dry with her sleeve. In this moment the dead lady is everything and Saint Nicholas is nothing. Nurse Snezhana Spazovska, Dr Aquarius, Sammy the driver; it's the longest I've seen them stay on scene. Never could I imagine that these hardened Macedonian medics on hearing this seemingly endless song would become so sad and – God forbid – weep. Nor could I imagine the gypsies of Shutka would appreciate our presence like they do now, our willingness to stay and listen, to give the most valuable gift a medic can give a patient – the gift of genuine feeling.

On the way back to Chaiar, Sammy gets us back in the mood with a disco-mix tape and cracks a few dirty jokes. It is 1 am when we pull into the ambulance station and I'm glad to have my feet on the ground again.

'Benja!' says Dr Aquarius, slapping me playfully on the way into the station. 'Seriously, you want to see Double Double X Irena? She is singing all night long!'

Sammy and Nurse Spazovska chuckle, but all I want to do is lie down.

'No? No, you're right. Double Double X Irena can wait,' she says, leading me through the door. It's at this moment that I see my worst nightmare. Resting on the table are three unopened bottles of Macedonian *rakija*.

'First, Benja, a little something to keep us going.'

ISLAND OF THE MONSTER WAVE

Thailand

Spectacular things may be beautiful and terrifying at the same time and so was the wave from which we ran. We ran as if pursued by a wild animal, while behind us, a wall of white water thundered through the palms, scattering a matchstick bungalow village and swallowing the flailing bodies of the Thai proprietors who had prepared our marvellous Christmas roast the night before.

A gentle shaking of our bamboo hut in the morning had woken Kass and me, but we thought little of it. A man brought us fresh juice that we sipped while taking in another cloudless sky over the shimmering Andaman Sea. It was then we saw the tide retreat as quickly as a drained bathtub. Out in the distance a line of pure white appeared across the horizon, approaching fast. The wonder of this enormous wave on a forever waveless expanse rooted us to the sand in total awe. Even as pandemonium broke out on the beach we stood there, completely under the spell of nature's might until the wave was nearly upon us. Then, as the tower of whitewash struck the shore, we turned on our heels.

Up the hill on the highest point of Koh Lanta we huddle with other backpackers, families and holidaymakers and locals, glancing down at the coastline with frightened eyes. Will there be another wave? Will it be larger still? Are we safe up here? Is it the end of the world?

Kass and I are in little more than our bathers and, like everyone else, we are stunned. Two days into our long-awaited holiday, and it's over.

'If only I had an ambulance now,' I say to her. 'I might be half useful.'

A young woman from Ecuador overhears me and tells us she is a medical student in her final year. Her name is Maria and together we canvass the rest of the people on the hill and find an ambulance officer from New Zealand by the name of Jimmy. Suddenly we have a medical team of sorts, without a bandage between us. We descend the hill to a road that circles the island, hoping to commandeer a vehicle. Kass somewhat reluctantly remains behind, taking care of those who have fled the coast. After almost a decade together, she is getting used to my disappearances in moments of crisis. She sighs at my every call to action, but never fails to send me off with a tender kiss. She's an artist, a designer, an entertainer who loves beauty and peace, yet has found herself too often in dangerous cities or witnessing disasters, thanks to her partner.

On the road our ragtag medical team doesn't wait long for transport. A utility pre-packed with injured Thais hurtles round the bend, barrelling down on us. We wave for it to stop and climb onto the back, stepping among a groaning pile of people clutching broken limbs and bleeding head wounds. Taking a left turn into the jungle, the utility begins traversing the centre of the island to a clinic on the other side. It's a dirt road of impossible potholes the driver takes at a speed more appropriate for German autobahns. We're tossed up and down as we attempt to assess the injured who shriek in pain at every jolt. Lacking our stethoscopes and blood pressure cuffs, we work with what we have. From experience I know that a patient with a strong radial pulse probably has an acceptable blood pressure for the time being and that breathing can be judged by placing an ear against the patient's chest. Most bleeding can be arrested with pressure, clothing can serve as pads and bandages, and opposing limbs make worthy splints. Indeed, when it comes to trauma, there is much that can be done riding in the tray of a makeshift ambulance without gear.

A neat lawn outside the Koh Lanta clinic is spread with victims of the tsunami, perhaps thirty or forty men, women and children waiting for treatment. Some roll around crying and appear in very bad shape. Others don't move at all.

It is not often that paramedics will lay eyes on a sight that truly takes their breath away, but it happens here.

Across the floor, and three-to-a-bed, are casualties with varying degrees of injury, sustained by the trauma of being lifted by the giant wave and thrown against buildings or trees or boats, tangled among heavy debris. The sleepy clinic would normally see no more than a few patients a day for coughs and colds, I suspect. Suddenly, with one doctor and couple of nurses, it has become one of the busiest trauma centres in the world.

Straddling a patient on the only resuscitation bed, a nurse is doing CPR on a young man covered in abrasions and deep, bleeding lacerations. The tall Thai doctor in charge of the clinic is wearing a clean white coat and is standing at the patient's head attempting to intubate, his eyes looking down the blade of an inserted laryngoscope.

We introduce ourselves and without looking up he says, 'Suction, suction, suction.'

Jimmy the New Zealand ambulance officer turns on the wall-mounted suction unit and hands the doctor a Yankaur sucker. After he slips it into the patient's mouth there is a steady slurping, much like the sound of a child finishing off a milkshake, and the perspex jar fills with blood. Already the doctor has placed bilateral chest tubes into the patient making it obvious he's no village GP. Although I do wonder about his decision in the face of such an extreme patient influx, to attempt the resuscitation of a traumatic cardiac arrest. I suspect the patient must have come in alive and gone downhill since.

'No good,' says the doctor, pulling out the scope. 'Here,' he thrusts the handle at me, ignoring the fact I'm in my swim shorts and looking like some sort of hippie surfer. Reluctantly I take the laryngoscope, slide it in and scoop aside the tongue, trying to make out the cords.

It's a total mess. Blood has risen past the man's epiglottis up into the mouth. Despite full suction, more blood appears, like a bottomless cup. Even with chest compressions I see no bubbles rising from the blood and my few blind attempts are futile.

Cardiac arrests following blunt trauma have close to zero chance of survival, according to my training in Johannesburg. Even at the best of times, with plentiful resources on hand, most emergency practitioners will avoid the charade of a resuscitation attempt. In the event of a disaster, it is particularly discouraged. When demand outweighs available resources, medics must revert to the principle of 'the greatest good for the greatest number'. Under normal circumstances, a non-breathing patient will get the undivided attention of at least two paramedics. But in the case of a disaster, the rules change. In disasters, once the airway is opened, if there is no breathing, we move on.

I shake my head and hand the scope back.

The nurse doing chest compressions stops and asks in English, 'What is on the monitor?'

We all look at the screen and see a green, unblinking line.

'Okay, finish,' says the doctor, glancing at his watch.

This we all think is a good idea. The nurse draws a sheet over the dead man's face.

'Any plans for evacuation?' I ask.

'They were busy last time we tried to radio.'

'I'll try Bangkok again,' says the nurse.

'Have you got a triage plan?' I ask the doctor.

He shakes his head. 'Not yet, no, we don't have. Can you manage it?'

Considering I wasn't able to 'manage' the intubation, I'm surprised the doctor wants me to triage. In the corridor, Maria is attending to a semiconscious villager dumped there by his friends. Beyond them, through the glass shutters to the driveway, I see more 'utility ambulances' arriving, their trays heaped with casualties. Rarely in my career have I had to deal with more than four or five patients at a time. In moments like this the word 'no', in any language, is cowardly.

'I'll do it,' I say, 'but I'll need blank paper and a pen.'

Without coloured triage tags I revert to a numbering system of one to four, one being the equivalent of red tags given to immediate patients, two in the place of orange tags for the serious but not immediately life-threatening, three for the green walking wounded and four representing white tags for the dead. The Thai doctor now works his way through the new casualties assisted by Maria, while Jimmy and I make a brief assessment of each patient and assign them a priority. Most of these patients are lying on blankets and sarongs spread across the floor due to lack of space and there is nothing much we can do about it. Most have fractures and nasty lacerations. Some are drowsy or amnesic after head trauma. One man is white and clammy and clutches a distended abdomen. He gets a 'priority one', as does another man semiconscious in the corridor.

The nurse returns and says, 'First helicopter coming in twenty minutes.'

This is excellent news as we imagine other islands have also been affected by the wave, though none of us are yet aware of how widespread and devastating it has truly been.

We are interrupted by horns beeping outside and glance up from our work to see a man scooping a young girl off the back of his pick-up truck. She is conscious, but her head is lolling round like a broken doll. He comes through the door and lies the girl at my feet and from his pained face I see he must be her father.

She is no more than twelve years old. Brushing the hair away from her face I reveal not one, but two black eyes that make her appear more like a victim of assault than a natural calamity. It's the first time I've seen such a definitive example of periorbital ecchimossis, the classic 'raccoon eyes' indicating a base of skull fracture. This would also explain her inability to maintain her head in an upright position. Bluish bruising known as 'battles sign' around the back of her head is the clincher.

'Jimmy, keep her still, hold her head,' I tell him. Then to the Thai nurse, 'Ask her father to continue reassuring her and can you bring a neck collar?'

By the time we hear the first military helicopter overhead we have five 'priority one' patients packaged and ready to airlift. Landing on a field hemmed in by jungle just behind the clinic, the chopper keeps its rotors running for a 'hot load'. Three Thai Air Force men remove a pallet of natural spring water and dump it on the grass. In return we stretcher our patients out and lie them directly onto the floor of the chopper, each beside the other. With no medic onboard it's a good thing the flight to Bangkok is a short one.

'We come back after dropping patients,' shouts a crewman above thundering rotors. 'Give us maximum one hour.'

The door slides shut and they lift off.

Back inside the hospital the Thai nurse tells me I have a phone call. I can't imagine who on earth it could be. When I go to the phone I hear my father's voice.

'Mate,' he laughs, 'thought you might be at the hospital over there. We'll let people know you're okay. Oh yeah, and Mum says make sure you wear sunscreen.'

A COUNTRY TO SAVE

Pakistan

The Khyber Road is near empty, the morning so crisp and fragrant with blossoming flowers that it's possible to imagine we are somewhere else, a mountain village of the Hindu Kush perhaps, anywhere but the city of Peshawar.

It is 2010 and few people know I'm here. My wife Kass and my family in Sydney would worry themselves silly if they found out. Officially, I'm in Pakistan to shoot footage of ambulances in Karachi and Lahore, not visit my old friends living less than thirty kilometres from the Afghan border. But the personable Vasif Shinwari, one of my fixers on *Son of a Lion*, a feature film I shot a few years ago in the area, insisted I spend a week with his clan, luring me with promises of meeting the director of emergency services at Lady Reading Hospital.

Peshawar is gripped with fear. Makeshift checkpoints have been set up on every main street and the police manning them visibly tremble as they stop each car. Suicide bombers, most thought to originate from the extremist outfit Tehreek-e-Taliban, based in Waziristan, have converged on the city, detonating every other day in response to the Pakistani Army's campaign against them. Hundreds of people in Peshawar have been killed as a result. Businesses and government buildings have been fortified with Hesco blocks and coils of barbed wire, and concrete barriers are set out on the street to prevent car-bombers from reaching targets. Any structure, vehicle or individual connected with either the government of Pakistan or a foreign nation is fair game.

Last night, when Vasif offered to take me on a tour of the blast sights in his new Land Rover I flatly refused. Vehicles like this are commonly driven by representatives of international NGOs or Pakistani officials and keenly targeted by suicide bombers.

'Don't worry,' he said in his brigadier's English. 'My baby is under the front seat.'

His 'baby', it turns out, was a fully loaded 20-shot sub-machine gun. It seemed an impressive weapon when he showed me, but I find little reassurance in the idea of a gunfight. Many recent attacks have involved teams of militants with hand grenades and explosives. Would Vasif and his 'baby' really come up trumps?

On our way to Lady Reading Hospital we pass the ruined Peshawar headquarters of Pakistan's spy agency, the Inter-Services Intelligence (ISI), demolished by a truck bomber the week before. Nervous sentries stand watch in the rubble. On the opposite side of the road, Peshawar's fairground with its lurid carousel is locked up as it has been for more than a year. When I express my disappointment to Vasif he wants to know if I think people need fun in a time of war.

'Why not?' I say. 'Isn't fun a healing thing?'

'Maybe, but like everything else in Pakistan, the fun park is owned by our army and that makes it a target.'

Further down the road towards the old city I point to an oddly shaped building painted in grimy pink where a large crowd is milling, pushing to get inside. Vasif tells me it's the judicial complex, the district courts where people come from all over the frontier to have their cases heard.

We drive on and cross the next set of lights. It's at this moment, less than thirty seconds after passing the judicial complex, that a suicide bomber detonates among the crowd behind us. Thinking the sound to be nothing more than a car backfiring we drive on oblivious, admiring the Bala Hisar Fort looming above and soon arrive at the hospital behind it. Here we realise something has happened. As we pass through the front gates the security guards are shouting at one another and porters are frantically rushing metal trolleys to the emergency dock. Walking briskly towards us is Vasif's friend, the Chief Medical Superintendent, Abdul Hameed Afridi, who confirms there has been another blast, this time at the judicial complex, and warns us to keep clear of the pandemonium about to ensue.

Hearing the wail of an approaching siren we know there is no time to reflect on our lucky escape. We head to the main ramp of the emergency ward as an old Suzuki ambulance bounces through the gates and skids to a halt. Opening the rear door of the van is unnecessary, as it is already up. An unconscious man covered in blood and soot is pulled out and thrown onto a trolley and rushed up the ramp into the emergency ward. As other ambulances begin to arrive they too have their back doors open. Either these old vans have universally faulty latches or closing the back door is considered a waste of precious time. Studying news footage of the judicial complex bombing the following day, I would see just how these ambulances end up transporting patients with the back doors open. While drivers appear to shut them before departing, the doors are inevitably wrenched open again by hysterical members of the public, eager to throw more victims in. This happens even as an ambulance is pulling away at speed. In Pakistan, the moment an ambulance arrives on the scene it becomes public property.

One by one they scream through the gates, news trucks too, along with crowds of spectators, until there is little room left for vehicles to turn around and head back out. From the sidelines, Vasif and I watch the gruesome delivery of casualties unloaded by a hundred hands. Many victims arrive with clothes torn off, limbs askew, hair and beards singed away. I can hear hearts break as a stone-faced father steps out of an ambulance holding the ragdoll body of his infant child. The crowd hushes for a moment and parts to let him through. Cameras flash furiously. Meanwhile, porters continue to wipe blood from trolleys with dirty rags ready for the onslaught of more ambulances.

Part of me wants to lend a hand, but there are so many volunteers already helping out it seems the entire city has turned up. This sense of community that ethnic Pashtuns are so famous for ensures no shortage of assistance.

An ambulance packed with walking wounded screeches in and I'm startled to see fatty chunks of indistinguishable human flesh rolling about at their feet. More disturbing still is the next vehicle containing a charred corpse shredded into strips followed by an ambulance carrying small packages of body pieces wrapped in towels, dripping blood and entrails as if scavenged from a butchery. Up the ramp it all goes, past surly security men who guard the entrance with electric cattle prods, zapping a throng of curious youth, concerned relatives and friends all trying to slip inside.

Among the drama, Vasif takes a phone call and I hear him reassure his wife Sheema we are both okay. Vasif's uncle, says Sheema, was playing golf at the time of the blast when a human arm landed on the green. So the fun park is closed but golf is okay?

Half an hour later we are in the office of Shiraz Afridi, head of the emergency department. He is the spitting image of the late Osama bin Laden and it is no wonder Afridi has, in the past, been routinely stopped by authorities on his way to overseas medical conferences. In contrast to the world's most formidable terrorist, Dr Afridi is among the most respected emergency physicians in Pakistan. He has US and Irish qualifications in disaster management and runs one of the busiest casualty departments in central Asia.

Seeing us come through the door, Dr Afridi gets up excitedly and smothers me in a hearty embrace, ordering his assistant to brew some tea. Right away one can tell he is a charismatic man, though it surprises me how relaxed he seems less than an hour after a barrage of trauma. He motions for us to sit and I sense he has read my mind.

'Taking tea is okay now, the rush is over,' he says, as two phones on his desk ring simultaneously. 'Excuse me for a second.' On one line he has the Pakistani Red Crescent whom he puts on hold to field an enquiry from CNN.

'Yes, so far we have more than fifty injured and nineteen expired … yes, nineteen, only. We are managing well, committed to easing the pain of our fellow Pakistanis, ready for anything, yes, thank you.'

Vasif excuses himself, says he will send his driver to pick me up later on. As he goes out, the chief surgeon drops by to inform Dr Afridi that one of the patients in theatre has just passed away during a chest operation, raising the death toll to twenty. Another man shuffles in with a stores order for him to sign while an anxious-looking gentleman who has made it past numerous security points stumbles through the door begging for a prescription to be filled. Graciously Dr Afridi scribbles something on a form and the man backs out, bowing repeatedly. Not once does the doctor lose his cool.

'You know, this was not a big blast. Last month, after the Meena Bazaar bombing, we got over a hundred expired and three hundred injured. That was a little more challenging. But our reflexes are quicker now due to this extra burden. A doctor in our emergency department can see six patients in the time a doctor in your country sees one. An average of 1500 patients a day come through here, even without a bombing. We have adapted to these war conditions. Until four or five years ago no one at Lady Reading had ever experienced the aftermath of a suicide attack. It is only a recent phenomenon in Pakistan. While foreign troops remain in Afghanistan we will continue to see this problem.'

I tell Dr Afridi about my interest in pre-hospital care and ask him about ambulances in Peshawar. Although the city has a small fleet of dented Suzuki vans, patients from surrounding villages usually arrive still lying on their own *charpoy* rope beds which relatives have carried in or loaded on the back of pick-up trucks.

'It's true to say much progress is required. As you have just witnessed, those ambulances outside belong to our national hero Abdul Sattar Edhi. They are fairly rudimentary, I mean, *very* rudimentary. But things are evolving. It is exciting. Punjab has a new service, Rescue 1122, which I'm eager to see introduced in this city.'

On an earlier visit to Pakistan in 2004, I'd briefly experienced both services in Lahore. The Edhi Foundation, the largest welfare organisation in Pakistan, allowed me to ride along with ambulance crews during the Independence Day celebrations, at which time I helped collect the crumpled body of a man fallen from the towering Minar-e-Pakistan. Around the same time I befriended Dr Rizwan Naseer, a former trauma surgeon launching the country's first modern ambulance system and was invited to help train two hundred paramedics. While Edhi ambulances are greatly respected and available countrywide, they are simple vans containing little more than a stretcher and, if lucky, a cylinder of oxygen. In contrast, Rescue 1122 would provide an emergency service offering advanced first aid. Although established four years ago, 1122 is still largely confined to the province of Punjab.

My specific intention on this visit is to meet Abdul Sattar Edhi, the founder of the organisation, in Karachi before travelling to the headquarters of Rescue 1122 in Lahore to see how far they have come. Dr Afridi seems pleased to hear this and asks me to pass on regards to his old friend Dr Naseer with whom he had completed his Masters of Surgery.

'Tell him I've set the groundwork for his move into the north-west,' says Dr Afridi with a cheeky wink. 'You see, not long ago I was travelling in a car with the Director-General of Health for the province when we came across a nasty road accident. A jeep had rolled down a steep embankment and a passenger was suffering a tension pneumothorax. I requested a knife and the crowd were shocked seeing me slice the man's chest to free the trapped air. When this was done, I turned to the Director-General of Health and told him he had just witnessed pre-hospital care. I think only then, seeing this, did he really understand the importance of an effective ambulance service.'

We break for prayers and Dr Afridi takes his time in the bathroom. When the tap stops running he emerges with wet sleeves and wet trouser legs.

'It is a requirement of my religion to be clean before prayer. According to Islam, I must not have even the smallest drop of another man's blood on my clothes.'

Dr Afridi's assistant has laid out woven plastic mats and he begins reciting the call to prayer with fingers at his ears. Hearing the opening *Allahu Akbar* I reflect on the sad irony that these words – God is great – are also the last to leave the lips of suicide bombers.

When prayers are done, a boy brings in plates of meatballs, hot *roti* and bottles of cola. Perhaps it is not the best topic over dinner but I'm curious to know how body parts are matched up after the Peshawar attacks. In Israel, a rescue and recovery organisation known as ZAKA – the Hebrew acronym for 'Identification of Victims of Disaster' – combed the scene of every bombing throughout the second *intifada* for the smallest fragments of flesh. According to Jewish customs, a body needs to be buried with all its parts, no matter how small. To achieve this end, ZAKA uses advanced forensic techniques like DNA testing. When I mention this, Dr Afridi seems a little annoyed.

'Of course Israel can afford these things. I too believe it is important to find body parts, but this hospital doesn't even have an MRI scanner, let alone DNA technology. It is a shame because I am a strict Muslim and I do feel strongly about this.'

Hayat Khan, my long-time friend from the tribal areas, who had once attended the Cadet College Kohat with Shiraz Afridi, told me the doctor had become ultra-religious only after leaving school. Despite his jolly energy and good humour, I'd noticed the man's beard to be shaved above the top lip, the classic hallmark of a particularly pious Muslim.

'When the bombings began I lost too much sleep over this dilemma. Some of my staff were putting random legs and arms together, severed heads with wrong torsos and so on. This made me angry and I consulted Islamic scholars around Pakistan about it. There was a large convention of *ulema* and I waited some time for the outcome. Finally, their decision, based on the holy books, was that we are permitted to bury just the torso, even if limbs are missing. So I was satisfied. By the way,' he says, 'how are the meatballs?'

At first I think he is being funny, that characteristic humour possessed by medics worldwide. But he looks at me with a genuine desire to know that his hospitality is in order.

I nod, 'Delicious.'

'You know, it is a great honour to wash a body. There is a particular way a body must be prepared in Islam, how the shroud must be wrapped. Some of my female staff were frightened by the condition of those who expired in the Meena Bazaar attack, children burnt like chickens and so on. But I told my staff about what is written in the Qur'an, that if you wash the body of a fellow human being, your own sins are washed clean. Now they all want to wash the bodies. Makes me wonder about the extent of their sins,' he says, this time with a playful smile.

Dr Afridi takes me on a tour of the emergency ward at midday and I'm baffled to see not a single bed occupied.

'Where are the fifty injured people?' I want to know.

'We have managed them, treated them, discharged them or sent them to the operating theatre and distributed them to appropriate wards. Why hold a patient in this emergency department? It is for emergencies! Once emergency is over, a patient has no place here.'

Dr Afridi's stunning logic amuses me greatly. How a hospital with zero government funding can boast a vacant emergency department just hours after a major incident is hard to fathom. I tell him about the long afternoons I routinely spend stuck at hospitals in Sydney, unable to move a patient off my ambulance trolley for lack of available space.

'Yes, I've worked in Scotland and I remember in the emergency ward it was often about which doctor or nurse is due for the next lunch break. Here, when we are busy, doctors voluntarily come from other departments to ensure all patients are cleared from emergency. They do not eat or drink until it is done. We have great sense of public service in Pakistan. Wages are secondary. In the case of a blast, you have seen for yourself just how many volunteers arrive to help. Sometimes we even turn them away.'

'But a starving doctor will hardly possess the clarity of thought required for the job,' I say. The fasting month of Ramadan in particular must be difficult, not eating before sundown, on even the busiest days.

'Those doing Allah's work are nourished by it,' replies Dr Afridi, 'and they do not feel as hungry as you may think.'

Calm has once again returned to the entrance of the hospital. An old man from a remote village is lifted off the back of a truck and carried in on his own bed. It's a novel approach hospitals in Western nations with their scarcity of emergency beds would do well to adopt.

Almost as an afterthought Dr Afridi says, 'And your system is so crippled by fear of litigation. In Pakistan there is no concept of negligence. If something goes wrong we just tell them it was Allah's will.'

Indeed, excessive thoroughness in the West – such as CT-scans for anyone who has fainted – combined with a rising barrage of patients presenting to hospitals with minor complaints, are more likely the root causes of bed-block than too many lunch breaks taken by staff.

A car with tinted windows pulls up and a kind-looking man in a sharp black suit, Ejaz Afzal Khan, the Chief Justice of Peshawar, steps out and greets Dr Afridi. He has dropped by to check on the condition of lawyers injured in the suicide blast and pay his respect to those who have died.

'People came because of injustice and received an even greater one,' he says with a breaking voice.

Vasif's driver arrives and I bid farewell.

'Another cup of tea?' asks Shiraz Afridi while embracing me. But I know these words are just his way of saying goodbye. Pashtuns are perpetually anxious to ensure their guests depart with the song of hospitality sounding in their hearts.

Out on the street people are making a wide arc to avoid our parked car. Stationary vehicles unattended may represent the next car bomb and the cranky owner of a chemist nearby complains we are bad for business. The bombings have brought Pakistan to its knees on every level. Much like the fight-or-flight response of the human body to an external threat, a society cannot heal or grow in times of war when self-preservation is the order of the day. No one can be educated when schools are shut. No one can eat or trade when they are in the lockdown of a curfew or fearing the next blast. Tough as these times may be, however, survival is in the Pakistani blood. Today the city of Peshawar and the medics at Lady Reading have pulled together in the aftermath of a suicide bombing with more efficiency and spirit than many nations could muster for an ordinary weekday.

When Khalid Ali, a cousin of my friend Hayat Khan, meets me at the Jinnah International Airport in Karachi he is holding a sign with *Bin Yameen* printed on it – an Islamified version of my first name intended to avoid unwanted attention. The precaution appears to have failed though, as a chubby man in a baseball cap and Coke-bottle glasses follows us to the car, walking a few feet behind in the most obtrusive manner, filming our conversation with his mobile phone. Irritated, I stop and spin around, demanding to know what he's up to.

'Sir, I am making call to Germany,' he protests, quickly putting the phone to his ear and hurrying away.

Khalid Ali laughs. 'That's what they call undercover. Why are these secret agents so stupid? Don't worry, no one can touch you.'

Since shooting *Son of a Lion* in the Federally Administered Tribal Areas (FATA) between 2005 and 2007, I've been extremely critical of the Pakistani Army for its ruthless bombing of Pashtun civilians along the tribal belt while the government continues to covertly support Taliban groups fighting in Afghanistan. As a vocal advocate for ethnic Pashtuns I did not expect to be in the government's good books and just about everyone strongly advised me not to visit the country again. Pakistan's Inter-Services

Intelligence (ISI) are well known for their false-flag operations – assassinations and bomb blasts that are blamed on the 'terrorists'. But any fear I had was outweighed by an appointment to meet the world's greatest living ambulance service executive.

In just over fifty years, Abdul Sattar Edhi has created a health and welfare empire like no other. His ambulance service boasts 1600 vehicles across the country and is listed in the *Guinness Book of Records* as the largest on earth. At most major intersections across Pakistan, Edhi's white ambulances can be seen parked ready to respond. They can also be summoned by dialling 115. The man is a household name, a champion of the poor, a role model for the young, a hero of the masses. While most famous for his ambulance service, Edhi's work also extends to social welfare, homes for the geriatric and the destitute, orphanages, clinics for women, maternity hospitals and adoption services managed by his wife Bilquis.

My arrival in Karachi coincides with the holiday of Eid al-Adha, a festival commemorating the willingness of Abraham to sacrifice his son as an act of obedience to God before being commanded to slaughter a ram instead. All over the Islamic world, sheep, goats, cows and even the occasional camel are sacrificed in honour. None of the meat goes to waste and most of it ends up donated to the poor. All year round generous donors in Pakistan drop off hundreds of goats to local ambulance stations, many built with a special animal enclosure. By the time Eid al-Adha comes around, Edhi has amassed a considerable herd for the slaughter.

The night before I go to stay with Edhi I'm put up at the Hotel Saddam, a ramshackle place with oval-shaped 1960s tinted windows and, to my great amusement, white bed-sheets with 'Queensland Health' printed on them. Over a mouth-watering dinner of tandoori chicken, hot *roti* and cardamom pudding in a local restaurant, I fantasise for a time about the thrilling life of an international linen smuggler.

Early the next morning I'm on a bus without windows to Mithadar, possibly the poorest of Karachi's inner-city localities. The bus is packed and I stand awkwardly with my luggage until a number of passengers sitting down reach up and take my bags onto their laps. I even permit a cripple in threadbare trousers to tenderly nurse my camera that costs more than he will earn in a decade. Many may call me a fool, but I sense this man would die before letting anything happen to my valuables, another moving reminder of how well the people of Pakistan treat their guests.

Streets around Mithadar bustle with donkey carts and tooting cars and people lugging unusual loads on their heads. It's the last day of work before Eid al-Adha and smoking coolies yell out as they drag overladen carts past grubby children playing cricket in alleyways with splintery planks. Tall Raj-era buildings look close to collapse in this densely populated neighbourhood where Abdul Sattar Edhi first opened shop in 1957. That was the year he bought a beat-up Hillman van for 7000 rupees – about US$100 – onto which he had painted the words 'Poor Man's Ambulance'. In no time he was operating the sole ambulance for a city of a million, sweating around the clock. In his 1996 biography, *Mirror to the Blind*, Edhi talks of the days he would drive the ambulance from one accident to another without a break until his 'head was spinning'. Of any living person, Edhi is thought to have gone the longest time without a holiday – seventy-eight years or thereabouts – calculated from the age of five when his mother inspired him to begin voluntary social work.

In his early days in Mithadar, Edhi retrieved drowned bodies from the sea, from rivers and from wells, bodies that broke apart with one touch. He picked them up from manholes and gutters, from under bridges and railway tracks. And no matter how infested with maggots or how decomposed they were, he brought them home and prepared them for burial.

The thought of hoisting a body three-weeks dead onto my

shoulders or collecting dismembered limbs without gloves has me cringing. But this, this revulsion I feel, is the very attitude that Edhi warns of in his book.

'We cannot truly reduce suffering,' he says, 'until we are able to rise above our own senses.'

Thanks to this strong stomach and iron spirit, Edhi is said to have prepared almost twenty thousand Pakistani bodies for burial with his bare hands.

Following a trail of dung and, soon after, a convoy of animals, I come upon the man himself sitting among a flock of grubby sheep some would consider unfitting company for the chief executive of an organisation worth a billion rupees a year. But Edhi owns little more than two sets of simple *shalwar kameez* – the traditional Pakistani long shirt and pants – eats one modest meal a day and for most of his life has slept on the cold floor of his office. It's precisely this self-imposed poverty that allows him to identify with those he helps.

On seeing me he stands up, an eighty-three-year-old man with a flowing silver beard. He pushes some of the flock aside and greets me with a customary hug and handshake before turning back to his animals. I suppose for Edhi I am just one of countless people who travel from afar to see him and I'm grateful his manager has told me I can stay as long as I like.

While Edhi's team of female assistants put the kettle on he remains in the street, and almost all who pass him stop and bow and take his hand or touch his feet in awe. Edhi accepts it all with a nod and the occasional twinkle in the eye. But when a mentally disturbed man arrives covered in dried excrement, pulling at his own hair and cursing to himself, Edhi breaks into a generous smile and is particularly happy. Though he claims to speak no English, he turns to me and says, 'This man, very love!'

Next is an ancient woman hobbling past, bent and gnarled, all her possessions wrapped in a small sackcloth bundle. Edhi clasps her hand then reaches into his pocket to retrieve a thick rolled wad of 1000 rupee notes from which he counts a few out for her. While Edhi has always dreamed Pakistan will become a modern welfare state, until that day comes, thousands remain dependent on this one man.

Seeing the old woman's luck, a much younger one with matted hair and grimy face approaches Edhi begging for cash but is sent reeling by a tirade of angry shouting. I notice Edhi has a tough exterior, much like the war-weary triage nurses I know back home who have plenty of patience for genuine cases but are intolerant of opportunists, hypochondriacs and troublemakers.

When the dust settles, Edhi beckons me inside for tea and I ask him about his activities over the holiday of Eid, while one of his assistants translates.

'Yesterday we sent 250 goats to Waziristan,' he says, referring to that troubled agency in the tribal areas where Pakistani forces are fighting America's war against Pashtun insurgents, killing and displacing thousands of civilians in the process. 'We escorted the goats in a fleet of ambulances. The ambulances too we left in the town of Wana for locals to call upon.'

Obsessed as I am with sterile working environments, hearing about the transportation of goats by ambulance has me feeling a little nauseous. Already I noticed the ambulance parked outside his office is filled with cattle feed. And now, as we take tea, the stench of sheep urine wafts through the open door. It's clear to me that Edhi has more important things to worry about than hygiene. Same goes for the condition of his headquarters, centre of the world's biggest private ambulance service. There are no computers and his logbooks and papers are stacked to the roof. Important phone numbers are scrawled directly onto the walls with black marker. But my journeys through developing nations have revealed that many of the most effective humanitarians are poor administrators and pathologically untidy, while the slickest aid organisations spend a criminal amount of donor money on unimportant things.

'We held a peace march in Waziristan, encouraging the Taliban to stop with suicide bombings. We told them not to spread religion through force and to convince people instead through good example.'

Over the past five years, hundreds of pro-peace tribal elders conveying the same message in FATA have wound up beheaded. Did Edhi not fear this would happen to him?

'Everyone has to die. If you feel fear you can't do anything, you are like a stone. Fear is an insult to God, that you don't trust His protection. Taliban pay respect to me anyway. They have good memory. They remember all the ambulances my men drove to Afghanistan after America's invasion, picking up the wounded *mujahideen*, repatriating them back across the Pakistani border.'

No wonder the Taliban hold him in high regard. Plenty may owe him their lives. Those injured fighters – likely to number in the hundreds – would have been eternally grateful to leave Afghanistan in a friendly ambulance rather than a US Air Force C-17 to Guantanamo, bag over the head.

'You love to blame the Taliban but much of this mess has been created by the government of Pakistan. They have forced Taliban out of the mosque to defend the ordinary people of the frontier who are under attack. Foreign nations support our criminal leaders while our common people fight for true justice. We have lost faith in the whole world.'

Edhi is never shy to speak his mind. In a country where journalists disappear or end up in jail for criticising the government, Edhi's popularity makes him untouchable. His reputation also allows him enviable access to areas where no one else can go. While countless Pakistani NGOs drool over $750 million of US aid money allocated for the tribal areas, most of it remains in the bank, gathering dust due to lack of security in

FATA and a shortage of reliable partners. While tragically ironic, Pakistan's most trusted individual and experienced humanitarian would never accept a single cent of US aid, despite being the best man to spend it. Abdul Sattar Edhi believes this kind of money is tied up in politics, the very politics responsible for creating such dismal conditions for Pakistanis in the first place.

A homely lady with long plaited hair enters the room. She adjusts her shawl when she sees me and gives a welcoming smile. Edhi's wife Bilquis is just as busy as her husband, supervising maternity clinics, nursing schools and adoptions services offered by the foundation. In his biography, Edhi admits that many of her friends warned her about marrying such a serious man bearing so much of society's pain and horror upon his shoulders. 'Our husbands will take us for picnics while yours will take you to graveyards! We will beautify ourselves while you will embalm and scent the dead!' Despite these predictions, the couple wed in 1966. Later, when I ask Bilquis if her friends had been right, she gives a cheeky smile and nods. It has taken her fifty years of marriage to convince Edhi that fun is not necessarily indulgent and that picnics are equally nourishing for the human spirit.

'Our first picnic was in 1973 on our Hajj pilgrimage. We drove an ambulance all the way to Mecca, nearly 3000 kilometres, stopping in the deserts along the way for roast chicken and watermelon.' Since then, Edhi enjoys a picnic. Nowadays he even arranges them on a regular basis for the disabled and terminally ill.

Upstairs Bilquis lays out a sumptuous lunch of lamb curries, saffron *biryani* and cucumber salad on a yellow tablecloth embroidered with flowers. I sit beside Edhi and break bread with him. Being in the presence of greatness has never felt so normal. Edhi connects directly with his followers and, at almost twenty years older than the accepted Western age for retirement, the man still responds to emergencies, his hands shaking with Parkinson's disease.

'Yes, on the day I die, you will find me in an ambulance,' he says, passing me a plate of sliced radish. 'How can I expect my staff to do the job if I am unable?'

Edhi has always led from the front. After Palestinian gunmen hijacked Pan Am Flight 73 in Karachi on 5 September 1981, he was the only one permitted on the tarmac and personally carried away the body of Neerja Bhanot, an Indian air hostess shot dead after challenging the hijackers. Most recently, when the dismembered remains of Wall Street journalist Daniel Pearl were found in a shallow grave north of Karachi, Edhi himself gathered up all ten parts and drove them to the morgue. Most would agree his mere presence is an honour to the sick, injured or recently dead.

A young boy with neat hair arrives carrying two bottles of Pepsi and pours me a glass. Even Edhi drinks some, explaining his new diet of meat and Pepsi comes on doctor's orders due to his failing health. Most of his adult life he has survived on dry bread and water alone in order to identify with the poor. It is the same concept as Ramadan.

'A full stomach teaches nothing,' he says.

The boy joins us and introduces himself as Saad, Edhi's eleven-year-old grandson. He has a pleasant face, soft features and kind eyes, the way I imagine Edhi might have looked as a child. It's a fitting comparison because Saad is set to inherit The Edhi Foundation and his grandfather has been grooming him from when he first started riding on ambulances at the age of eight. While Edhi is likely to be the world's oldest ambulance worker, Saad is no doubt the youngest. Together they have travelled all over the state of Sindh and beyond, pulling rotten bodies from ditches, men hanging from trees or caught in the crossfire of police battling *dacoits*. While parents in the West try to shield their young from horrors of the world, Edhi sends his grandson down wells to retrieve dead babies.

Between mouthfuls of rice, Saad winds a fluorescent plastic watch on his wrist and I see the child in him. He is shy and softly spoken. When I ask if it bothers him growing up surrounded by so much sadness, he shrugs and is unnecessarily modest.

'It's nothing,' he replies in English. I wonder if he is putting on a brave face in the presence of his grandfather.

'Have you counted the number of bodies you've seen?' I enquire, catching myself asking him the most clichéd and irritating question one can put to an ambulance worker. But Saad doesn't seem to mind.

'Yes, so far I count one-hundred-and-fifty.'

'He's only young, you know,' laughs Edhi dismissively at what he evidently regards a petty number.

Slowly all over the city muezzin calls spring up from speakers on buildings, poles and mosques until the air is dancing with a thousand crackly voices. Saad excuses himself and performs ablutions in a sink by the door, closely followed by his grandfather. The boy rolls out a woven mat and pulls up a chair for his elder, a man so riddled with arthritis he can no longer prostrate himself. For twenty minutes during *dhuhr* prayers I observe the two of them meditating side by side, the past and the future hope of Pakistan's poor, under the blessed gaze of Allah.

That evening at an intersection miles from Mithadar, I shell peanuts with Edhi's ambulance drivers and wait for a call. The streets are frantic and clouds of exhaust glow in the blinking carnival lights of Karachi's festooned buses, rising around men in billowing *shalwar kameez* running to catch them. Women wait to cross the road, covered from head-to-toe in black *chaddars* rendering them almost invisible in the disappearing light, children clutched to their sides, bags of shopping on their heads. Among the bustle, a little boy sells goldfish in plastic bags of fresh water, his small, fragile voice ringing out across the noise.

There are fourteen emergency posts like this across Karachi, single-room concrete structures with space enough for two or three people to sit down. We choose to remain outside inhaling the fumes and atmosphere of a Pakistani peak hour, swapping stories. One young man named Rahul tells me he was first on the scene of Benazir Bhutto's homecoming bomb blast in October 2007 which killed 130 people and injured three times that number.

'Everyone wanted my ambulance,' he says. 'In seconds the worst injured you can imagine were inside. Each time I went back for more my ambulance was filled with the dead. That night I set personal record of fourteen bodies and many extra body parts all inside my ambulance at once.'

Having witnessed Edhi ambulances in Peshawar less than a week ago, I can picture it well.

'Generally,' he continues, 'I will try not to make a bundle of injureds.'

Tales of exploding ordnance factories with hundreds of people wounded, packed buses crashing off flyovers and mass drowning cases at Karachi's Clifton Beach make it difficult for me to compete with stories of assisting elderly ladies off the floor in suburban Sydney. Sitting there on a hardwood bench outside a filthy shack by the roadside, I wow them instead with descriptions of opulent ambulance stations in the West, stations with plush carpets, cable televisions, gymnasiums, pool tables and reclining lounges. Tell us more, they beg, tell us everything! So I show them a photo in which I'm standing beside an ambulance with my colleagues in Sydney, our uniforms pristine white, encircled by state-of-the-art equipment. In contrast, these men wear fraying *shalwar kameez* pyjamas with poor quality reflective vests that don't reflect, sewn by Bilquis Edhi herself on her old Singer. Buying the real deal from overseas was considered a financial indulgence by Edhi, money unnecessarily wasted in the face of the poor.

A few kilometres up the road a gas cylinder has blown apart and there are multiple casualties. Rahul drives madly, pounding the horn and siren, lane-splitting dense traffic, desperate to meet Edhi's promised response time of three minutes. This standard is probably one of the most impressive I've come across and although I doubt somewhat the reliability of the data, having Edhi outposts at every accident black spot means the service is remarkably prompt. Given that health ministries around the world judge response times to be the most important key performance indicator (KPI), the Edhi Foundation would rank pretty highly.

People scatter in our path and I genuinely fear we will kill or be killed. Rahul catapults our van towards the incident with complete disregard for safety. As a result of the holiday traffic we arrive fifteen minutes later to find most of the critically injured have already departed on local rickshaws. Only those with minor injuries remain but our ambulance is ill-equipped to offer anything but transport. It's 2009 and many of Pakistan's urbanites have made considerable progress in terms of business, quality of life and expectation of services. I wonder how long Edhi is able to rely on his rapid response times and urgent transport to satisfy the public. Already in the neighbouring province of Punjab, more sophisticated emergency medical services are being offered and embraced by a significant majority. Would it not make sense for Edhi to do the same, to update, advance, improve with the times?

It's now midnight and too late to bunk down on Edhi's floor as planned. Rahul takes me back to the Hotel Saddam instead and does this 'on the whistle', cranking the siren as we fly. Embarrassed, I obscure my face from the many heads turning to watch us pass, probably imagining we are off to some terrible tragedy. Unauthorised use of warning devices back home is a serious offence. Gone are the days when famous figures such as Orson Welles in New York owned personal ambulances for getting to appointments on time.

When Rahul skids to a halt outside my hotel I grab my bags and jump out, rushing into the foyer as if attending some critical case.

Rivers of blood course down tangled passageways of Mithadar early the next morning as Edhi's ambulance staff carve up hundreds of animals for Eid al-Adha. To reach the foundation's office I step over gaping goat heads, shanks piled high and a pyramid of discarded stomachs and hides. Carcasses lie everywhere while the massacre continues. Sheep and goats and some of the most enormous cows I've ever seen struggle against the ropes and weight of the humans holding them down. Thirty or forty onlookers have formed to watch five cows have their throats slit. I've enjoyed many a beef burger in my time but have never witnessed a cow's final moment. Children shriek as the giant creatures throw back their heads and spray arterial blood across their audience. Only when fully drained do the animals' eyes cloud over and legs stop kicking.

Against the wall of the dispensary a dozen of Edhi's ambulance drivers sit on straw mats with wooden chopping boards, made from the cross-sections of trees, wedged between their knees. Up and down their machetes go, the *chuck-chuck-chuck* of meat being diced. Mounds of steaming beef and mutton rise around them, while other men gather it up and into giant steel tubs that they carry to a storeroom for later distribution. Directing all this action is Edhi, shouting angrily, arms pointing this way and that, whacking one of his men on the shoulder, stopping only briefly to give me a wave.

By 9 am a steady stream of volunteers has begun to arrive. Once some paperwork has been signed they are given plastic bags filled with meat for delivery to designated slums and poor families around Karachi. Scavengers and beggars emerge from the shadows to try their luck but are chased away by Edhi wielding a stick as big as a police *lathi*. Edhi may seem prone to foul moods, allowing his detractors to label him a grumpy old man, but to me it is simply that he doesn't take bullshit.

Bilquis brings a bowl of fried liver pieces down from the kitchen so succulent and delicious I could scoff the lot. Pretending to hog the bowl, I cause one of Edhi's assistants to break out in giggles. On hearing this Edhi shouts at her to keep quiet. He snatches a cow tail off the ground and chases her squealing around the office. Failing to swat her, he tosses the tail on his desk and I detect an unmistakable playfulness in his eyes. It's clear that his temper is nothing more than a tool for his work.

'Come!' demands Edhi, motioning for me to get up as one of the girls helps him to a waiting ambulance. I climb into the back with the crew, squeezing myself between eight baskets of freshly chopped meat resting on the stretcher and floor. In no time we are off, lights and sirens wailing through the empty city, out into the sprawling settlements. I am finally riding in a true 'meat wagon' – that 1920s colloquialism for an ambulance.

Thanks to our siren the people of the settlements hear our approach a mile off and I see them running excitedly behind us. By the time we arrive at the community meeting hall, the ambulance is surrounded by a drooling mob. As I help lift a few baskets out, the crowd pounces, scrabbling for meat in utter desperation. Adults and teenagers throw each other aside to get their share. Small children dart like squirrels between the legs of the adults, retreating with little armfuls of flesh. Edhi calmly supervises the rush and in under a minute everything, down to the very last morsel, is gone.

At 'Tower Station', the busiest Edhi post and control centre where emergency calls are received and allocated, Edhi's ambulance staff lounge about on broken plastic chairs, a ragtag posse of betel nut-chewing characters with toothpicks behind their ears. Coughing and snorting and occasionally spitting fountains of bright red *pan masala* juice into the gutter, these ambulance workers hardly inspire one to call them in a crisis. Some hurriedly extinguish cigarettes under their dusty thongs when they see Edhi getting out of the ambulance, fearing his wrath. These are, however, the habits of the type Edhi has employed. How could the man possibly have found squeaky clean professionals for a job scooping up the shredded remains of blast victims with their bare hands. After all, latex gloves do not fit with Edhi's ideological opposition to 'cringing'. A barrier between rescuer and victim is a barrier between humans and God.

Edhi introduces me to Anwar Kazmi, his gaunt and toothless secretary of ambulance-related matters for more than forty years. In the Queen's English Kazmi offers me a rickety swivel chair and a dainty floral teacup of steaming *chai*. Sitting beside him is the secretary's secretary, a midget with thalidomide arms, his miniature legs crossed comfortably. All around us a veritable selection of grossly disfigured men with hunchbacks and malformed limbs shuffle away quietly, answering phones, filing papers, operating the ambulance dispatch. It's as if I have landed in the company of PT Barnum and his sideshow. Kazmi explains that Edhi is one of the few in Pakistan to employ the hideous and disabled. Many have grown up in the care of his orphanages, having been abandoned by their parents as infants. Handpainted signs on wrought-iron cradles permanently positioned outside every ambulance station in Pakistan read 'Do Not Kill Your Baby' – as innocuously as 'No Smoking' – and Edhi has received more than fifteen thousand children anonymously placed by night, many severely handicapped.

'All these men are committed to Edhi for life; he is their father,' Kazmi says.

Once upon a time, when Edhi began to expand, he and Kazmi attended accidents together, those glory days when the absence of any other ambulance service made them kings of the road. Nowadays, with American television shows and movies cabled into many Pakistani homes, people are well aware of what an ambulance should be. Have times changed for The Edhi Foundation? Are they feeling any pressure to modernise their vehicles, provide first-aid equipment and clinically competent medics? Are these not the fundamentals of pre-hospital care? After all, it is widely recognised that treatment *before* and *during* the journey to hospital have a drastic impact on survival.

Kazmi shrugs off these questions. 'People expect nothing in Pakistan. They understand we are a poor nation.'

Hearing my question, Edhi comes over to interrupt the conversation, obviously irritated. Kazmi translates for us while working his thumb around a rosary strand.

'All this talk of luxury ambulances!' Edhi snaps. 'Luxury is unavailable in a population where most people can't even get basic care. You say our population wants modern things. I say maybe one per cent don't like our standards, but 99 per cent need them. Our goal is the majority and a rich man will have to make do with the same ambulances that carry the poor. The truly suffering do not demand luxury.'

Perhaps he is right, although he never mentions the rapidly growing middle class in Pakistan numbering well over 30 million. As for those living below the poverty line, the most recent figures put this at 20 per cent, which may be far removed from Edhi's statistics, but is a considerable number nevertheless in a population of 168 million. Shoddy ambulances and unqualified staff may be of little concern to this group, but segments of Pakistani society do expect better, and some of these have told me they would rather take a taxi to hospital than a bone-jarring Edhi ambulance.

'What about Rescue 1122?' I ask him. 'They are now expanding to all of Punjab, offering a modern service, even to the poor.'

'So they say,' replies Edhi, clearly unconvinced. 'They're a government service. Look at me, I'm an old man with plenty experience and I can tell you the government of Pakistan has failed the people time and again. If Rescue 1122 saves lives, then this is a good thing. But let's see if they will last another five years, another change of government. Great ventures conceived by political parties are always shallow in this country. Our service, on the other hand, has weathered every political storm for sixty years.'

Anwar Kazmi wants to reassure me about the organisation's developments in training, informing me that Faisal Edhi, one of Edhi's sons, has recently returned from Europe where he qualified in disaster management.

'Already we are teaching our staff the concept of triage,' he says, beaming proudly. And about time too, I think. Almost a century has gone by since the term was coined. Having observed an Edhi crew in Peshawar transporting live and dead patients in a single ambulance, along with random body parts, made it obvious to me this area of training requires urgent attention.

'You see, our crews tend to pick up the dead people first. You must agree, they usually look worse off.'

We chuckle together.

Modernising vehicles and equipment is relatively easy if the funds exist. Harder, however, is the training of staff. Edhi's ten thousand drivers across Pakistan have little or no high school education, and many are illiterate. Such an employee profile would make reform a near impossible task without causing massive unemployment. Attracting high school and university graduates is unlikely when the average wage of an Edhi ambulance driver is 7000 rupees, about US$100 a month. This is less than half of what the new service Rescue 1122 pays its staff in Punjab.

Edhi is not alone in this dilemma. Many large EMS services in the USA, Europe and Australia faced the same problem in the early 1970s when men who were initially trained as drivers were pressured into qualifying as ambulance officers, some even as advanced paramedics. Due to rapid developments in pre-hospital health science and a greater public demand for paramedics on every ambulance, services continue to introduce extra skills, frequently above-and-beyond the abilities of their staff and without proper recompense. For Abdul Sattar Edhi such reform would be on a scale so great and of such impracticality and cost that his reluctance to entertain the idea of change is unsurprising. But with little concept or expectation of pre-hospital care, the poor in their millions continue to call him, as will all of those who have no alternative.

Edhi is often regarded as 'the Mother Teresa of Pakistan' and that comparison seems appropriate. At the age of nineteen I volunteered at Kalighat, Mother Teresa's home for the dying and destitute. My duties were to bathe old men encrusted with the filth of Calcutta, force-feed the malnourished and pick maggots out of open sores. It was challenging work. I feel the criticisms proferred by Mother Teresa's detractors are based on Western comparisons with some ideal that for most Indians living below the poverty line is simply unattainable. As long as a patient's condition is not made worse, 'something' is always better than 'nothing', and until the poor have free access to health care and are well informed about it, humanitarians like Mother Teresa and Edhi will step in with elementary services that will be gratefully accepted.

In his biography, Edhi has a clear message for those who point out his failure to progress: 'If these critics cannot share even a portion of their wealth with the poor, they should stop attacking me for sharing my poverty with them.'

President Zardari's seven-star hotel casts a tall shadow across the grey sand of Karachi's Clifton Beach, a testament to what is so sick about the country's ruling class and why millions of ordinary

Pakistanis continue to suffer.

It's Sunday and Sheroz, an Edhi ambulance driver, is accompanying me along the crowded boulevard past vendors selling garish shell souvenirs and groups of young men doing head-spinning dance routines. We stop here and there, once to have our photo taken with a cardboard cutout of Bollywood bombshell Aishwarya Rai and another time to drink from a fresh coconut split by a British-era sword.

Parking an ambulance by the seaside seems a universal distraction between emergency jobs, but I can't help reflecting on the contrast between the beaches of Clifton in Karachi and Bondi in Sydney. Here, waves of excrement roll onto a shore encrusted with litter where fully clothed men wander about aimlessly with pinky fingers linked. There is not a bikini in sight and I can only imagine what would happen to the first woman trying one out.

Swimming in the sea at Clifton Beach is equally hazardous and few people are daring enough to dip more than their feet. Sheroz insists he has swum here on many occasions and I'm not surprised, as a little later he tells me about plastic-bagging a man's brain earlier in the week after the poor chap was hit by a truck. Sheroz says he did this without gloves and, in his own words, 'even Dettol we not have'. What then is a bit of feculent seawater for a man who can stomach such a thing?

Sheroz goes on to explain how hazardous using gloves can be and I'm unsure I've heard him correctly.

'Yes, when we get to accident in poor and dangerous areas, people are seeing us with gloves and accusing us of acting like doctors. They attack us for being frauds. It is very confusing for them. They have no education about such things. Same is for first aid. Once I tried putting bandage on heavily bleeding patient and people started slapping me on head, yelling me to drive, just drive to the hospital, you idiot! What you think you are? Doctor? Drive! So the patient bled to death in the back. That is how the people are thinking. In very poor communities they do not understand.'

Rapidly forming mobs after accidents are not unique to Pakistan and I've seen a number of these while travelling through equally poor nations. If delaying transport to splint a leg or collar a neck risks being set upon by an angry and ignorant horde it is no wonder Edhi drivers prefer a rapid 'load and go' approach. This is another valid reason why Edhi himself is in no hurry to train his staff in pre-hospital care, not when the very action of applying first aid to patients can put them at risk of a lynching.

As if this is not enough danger for Pakistani ambulance workers, Sheroz tells me about a roster he recently did in the Swat Valley, a district in Khyber Pakhtunkhwa, the former North-West Frontier Province (NWFP), before the Pakistan military onslaught. Headless bodies of alleged spies were frequently found lying at traffic intersections during this time, placed there by militants to invoke fear in the population. According to a Taliban acquaintance of mine, it is far easier to shoot someone than behead them, but decapitation has a distinct political advantage. 'If you shoot sixty men, one may learn a lesson,' he told me. 'But if you behead one man, sixty learn it.' For full impact a headless body must therefore be 'on display' for as long as possible and in a prominent location. The problem for Sheroz and his colleagues called in to remove these bodies were the notes they found pinned to the clothes of the dead men.

'What was written on them?' I ask Sheroz.

'Do not pick. If you pick, we will kill you.'

Considering the number of police and army personnel kidnapped and murdered by militants around the province and knowing their every move was being watched by Taliban, Sheroz would give bodies a couple of hours in the street before carting them off.

On our way out of Clifton a man up ahead is hosing down the

road dust with a long pipe. As we pass by, water splashes up through my open window and onto my face. Sheroz sees this and passes me a box of scented tissues resting on the dashboard.

I shake my head and decline the offer.

'Never mind, it's only water,' I say.

'Ah, no sir, actually it is sewage.'

Disgusted, I take the box of tissues.

Sheroz answers a call on the radio and we begin driving around Karachi from one car accident to another. As we go, my colleague encourages me to take command of the handset controlling the megaphone speaker attached to the roof of the ambulance, which I accept with relish. So often we have longed for such a thing back home, less for the purpose of pushing through traffic than for the sheer amusement of broadcasting provocative comments and wolf-whistles to passing girls. As we hurtle like maniacs around Karachi, my voice is louder than the siren, my English seeming, in most cases, effective enough.

'MOVE LEFT! AMBULANCE PASSING! LEFT! LEFT! NO, *OTHER* LEFT! HEY, YOU WITH THE MOUSTACHE, MOVE LEFT!'

On one occasion we are beaten to the scene by a couple of other ambulance companies, all with equally poor vehicles and facilities but decorated as flamboyantly as Mister Whippy vans. One of them has the name CHHIPA stencilled on the side with a three-foot picture of some man's face bearing a mobster-like expression. The other belongs to an organisation known as KKF and instead of one grinning face it has three, all looking equally untrustworthy. Sheroz and his colleagues ignore these ambulances completely and we simply gather whatever casualties are left.

After the case, while eating sweet apples at a modest Edhi post on the outskirts of town, Sheroz expresses his frustration with the other ambulance companies.

'All of them belong to political parties. It is common practice now for political parties to start ambulance service in some part of the city as way of advertising. They drive around with sirens and everyone looks at them and sees what good work the political party is doing for the people.'

According to Sheroz, this disturbing political strategy is particularly prevalent in the state of Sindh, where every major incident or disaster is well covered by Karachi-based TV news cameras broadcasting around Pakistan and the world. Ambulances emblazoned with logos and images of political candidates have become an extremely effective tool for campaigning. Recently, on 19 October, Sheroz found himself in a squabble with drivers from CHHIPA over bodies recovered from an underground food storage facility where fifty women had been crushed to death in a stampede.

'It was terrible, these men arguing over the bodies of dead women, just so politicians can get their faces and banners on the evening news.'

For my last night with Edhi crews in Karachi, the control tower has sent three spare ambulances across town to try and find me some camel meat. Foolishly I'd admitted never having tried it. In the meantime, an Edhi driver with thirty years' continuous service pops a bottle of Pepsi for me and wipes the top of it with his greasy fingers. Reminding myself again about the lack of soap in the toilets, I'm overcome by a wave of nausea imagining the man has failed to properly wash his hands since the last body he delivered to the morgue. Considering their meagre wages, Pepsi is a beverage few drivers would ordinarily indulge in. For a celebratory bottle like this they would all have contributed their precious rupees and I know just how rude it would be to refuse drinking it on account of the germs awaiting my lips.

'Tell me, sir,' begins Sheroz. 'You know we go to many car accidents and injureds here in Karachi, so what kind of emergency do you attend in your country?'

Three other curious drivers huddle in for the answer.

'In my area,' I tell them, 'many people call because they are feeling anxious or depressed.'

A murmur rumbles through the group and there is head-shaking all round. Such incredulity is understandable considering Edhi drivers are used to severe trauma and death.

'Are you telling truth?'

'Of course, depression is no joke.'

Silence falls for a moment before Sheroz comes out with a corker and sends me reeling. In complete seriousness he asks, 'If people call you because they are in a sad mood, do they also call you when they are feeling romantic?'

Man, how I wish they would! If attractive romantics were making the calls, I dare say not another paramedic would complain about having their nightshifts interrupted.

At the Hotel Saddam later that evening I finish reading Edhi's biography and reflect for a time on its title, *A Mirror to the Blind*. I decide it refers to Edhi as the mirror and the rest of us as the blind. By looking at him we are able to see how oblivious we've become to the needy in our midst. Lack of luxury and pre-hospital medical care aside, it remains that Edhi guarantees an ambulance to anywhere in Pakistan within minutes. Furthermore, studies in America a decade ago suggest that in many cases of trauma there is marginal difference in patient outcomes between load-and-go transport and emergency care on scene. While anecdotal evidence contradicts these findings, there remains at least some scientific support for Edhi's claim that urgent transport by his ambulance drivers may indeed have saved millions of lives without any first aid whatsoever.

Given his lifelong dedication to the poor, the elderly, the outcast and orphaned, how blind we would be to have anything but praise for a man like Adbul Sattar Edhi.

On a humid morning filled with the sound of a thousand buzzing rickshaws, I'm escorted through the gates of the Rescue 1122 headquarters in Lahore under the watchful eyes of snipers and walk straight into an important board meeting of the service's newly appointed managers. There are thirty-six of them, one for each district of Punjab. I see the party are all turned out in their finest forest-green uniforms – the colour of the Prophet Mohammed, Peace Be Upon Him – pressed and decorated with sparkling stars and badges and names embroidered in silver thread. As I'm ushered in they rise from their seats and salute me. At the front of the room the iconic Director of Rescue 1122, my long-time friend Dr Rizwan Naseer, grasps my hand warmly and beckons me to sit beside him.

'Glad you could make it,' he grins.

Dr Naseer motions for the rest of the group to be seated before welcoming me as their honourable guest. Many of the men and women now holding senior management positions were among the first batch of paramedics I helped train in 2004 after I was introduced to Dr Naseer by the medical superindendent of Mayo Hospital near the old Walled City. All of them distinctly remember one lecture in particular.

'Ladies and babies!' squeaks a moon-faced manager. How could I forget the lesson that Dr Naseer had personally asked me to deliver? Obstetrics and gynaecology, a module no other trainer was game enough to attempt. Apart from one or two women, the first class of medics was overwhelmingly male. It should be noted here that these men reside in a country where the word 'girlfriend' is non-existent. Pakistani males in urban areas generally tie the knot late, hoping to be well established in business before embarking on marriage. Most will only ever experience the body of one woman, their wife. And even this, I'd been told, is usually done with the lights out. As for childbirth, men are rarely involved anyway. Dr Naseer had warned me at the time of my lecture that the subjects of birth and female anatomy were 'hidden things' in Pakistan and men were 'very reserved about womenfolk'. But taboos beckon to be broken, the forbidden breeds the curious, and the students hung on my every word. Since then, Dr Naseer has recruited several thousand more paramedics and suddenly I dread that he's been awaiting my return for a much bigger session on the same hot topic.

One by one the Rescue 1122 managers stand up to introduce themselves and convey the qualities of each Punjabi district they represent. Syed Qama Abid, a short gentleman with an impeccable moustache, announces in a horse jockey's voice he is the District Emergency Officer in charge of Sialkot District.

'Ah!' I say. 'The famous city of footballs!'

This acknowledgement of Sialkot's sports equipment industry delights him.

'Yes! Yes!' he chuffs. 'Sir, when I reach back to Sialkot, *inshallah*, I will send you a pair of finest soccer balls!'

Following the meeting, Abid gives me his visiting card with the words 'President's Gold Medallist' printed boldly under his name; an award he says is given annually to the 'best Boy Scout in Pakistan'.

The rest of the district managers are of equally fine stock, most being former military doctors poached from Pakistan's armed forces. In no time I've collected a veritable wad of visiting cards, perhaps the most important status symbol in a province where everyone seems to be desperately competing for importance.

Dr Naseer's office in a spacious front room of the grand nineteenth-century HQ is a shrine to the rescue and firefighting services he introduced to the country. Hundreds of plaques and badges, certificates and awards, trophies, medallions, framed newspaper spreads, and a gallery of ceremonial and hand-shaking photographs decorate the walls. Here, and at every ambulance station in the province of Punjab, hangs a three-foot portrait of Rescue 1122's baby-faced founder in full fire-resistant attire, nursing a polished black helmet in his right arm. Though it may seem self-aggrandising, I'm more inclined to view his portrait as essential strategy. Because Pakistanis love supporting a hero, a clever man will harness this passion, exploiting it for the purpose of his good works. The bearded face of Abdul Sattar Edhi is plastered on banners all over the country with pleas for donations – even the illiterate can respond to this visual symbolism. It is effective across every class and level of education. Followers of movements around the world acquire great strength from gazing at the spiritual leaders of their cause. And from what I can tell, Rescue 1122 has become such a movement in Pakistan.

'As you can see, much has changed!' he beams proudly. 'From our humble beginnings, a pilot project with no wages, and now this – seven thousand rescuers covering all of Punjab, population more than eighty million!'

Starting a free public ambulance service from scratch is no simple venture, least of all in a country as bureaucratically obstructive as Pakistan. The many obstacles such as gaining support from government, passing of new legislation, the massive set-up costs, ongoing funding, land acquisition, insurance, recruitment and clinical training, public access and education – let alone winning over the greater medical community – makes such a venture seem ludicrous for even the most ambitious individual. But as a leading orthopaedic surgeon with his own private hospital, Dr Naseer had become convinced that pre-hospital care was the missing link in the management of trauma and that if introduced it would greatly reduce morbidity and mortality among accident victims he was seeing. Motivated by a personal desire to improve the lives of his fellow Pakistanis, he expanded his knowledge of rescue and firefighting overseas before returning to Lahore with a plan. Supportive in principle alone, the Health Ministry had made clear to Dr Naseer they would wait until the service was fully functional and accepted by the people of Lahore before allocating funds. Enormous personal sacrifices were made by Dr Naseer in the first year as he relinquished his successful practice in Garden Town and piled millions of his own rupees into the pilot. But he was not the only one to suffer in the initial stages. The first two hundred recruits were employed under deferred-pay agreements and some complained to me in whispers how difficult it was providing for their families. Others even wondered if they were being taken for a ride. Dr Naseer continually urged patience, reassuring his staff that things would change once Rescue 1122 proved itself.

A few weeks later, on the first day of operation, the service faced an unprecedented demand. Emergency dispatch lines were jammed with calls for assistance and the new recruits were run off their feet. Within weeks the new rescue medics had become the heroes of Lahore. For the first time in years, media outlets heaped praise on the government of Pakistan for its initiative. The government took full credit for the service's development and, seeing a clear political benefit from its continuation, ordered the Ministry of Health to make a long-term financial commitment to keep it going.

Dr Naseer presses a switch on his table linked to a bell outside. Minutes later a boy rushes in with a tray of lunch. We tear off *roti* and scoop mutton curry into our mouths, washing it down with steaming glasses of Lipton tea.

While discussing service infrastructure, I'm struck by

the unique access I've been granted and the absurd degree of ceremonial respect I am lavished. At every turn I'm saluted like royalty, driven around and waited upon. It's embarrassing. But what is more embarrassing is my recollection of the day Dr Rizwan Naseer's own request to visit the Ambulance Service of New South Wales in 2005 was rejected. The superintendent in charge of foreign visitors at the time told me the service only offered tours to delegates of 'approved ambulance services'.

Bulletproof confidence is the key to strong leadership in Pakistan, but when Dr Naseer speaks about hurdles the service has faced in its first five years, he opens up to me in a way I doubt he would with his management team or road crews. To his staff he is a deity, a God-man gazing down from that portrait at every ambulance station. But with me it is different. Perhaps it's because I'm a friend who was there with him as he laid the earliest foundations of the service in 2004, discussing the way forward over long dinners at the Lahore Country Club, a posh British-era venue where guests are invited to experience the 'soothing effect of greenery'. Or perhaps it is because I'm an outsider harking from a nation where managers are considered 'only human'. Whatever the reason, Dr Naseer freely offloads years of frustration.

'It has been a constant struggle. First we had major dispatch problems, lines jammed from nuisance calls, hoaxers, pranksters, time-wasters. Mobile phone shops around the Punjab were making habit of testing new phones by dialling 1122. In early days we were getting a call every second of the minute. It was so bad that many people who really needed ambulances could simply not get through.'

'So what did you do?'

'We blocked all these calls. If the caller is not genuine, our system automatically bars that number in future. I know it seems unkind, but it is the boy-who-cried-wolf situation.'

'And if they have a real emergency?'

'Yes, sad to say it, but they may expire. It is their choice. We have publicised this fact, that if people want to make mischief, they will potentially suffer in future.'

'Is this the only controversy?'

Dr Naseer laughs.

'Always I am tied up with some drama. Last one was a claim made in *The Nation* newspaper that I am an infidel, a non-Muslim because I ban my staff from having beards. Some disgruntled ex-employee lodged an official complaint against me. This was very upsetting. All I ask of my staff is not to look like a *dacoit* or terrorist. It is very important in these sensitive times to protect our image when we attend blast sites and so on.'

'Did someone get fired?'

'Yes, but I tell you, not because of the beard. They used this fact as an excuse. It was matter of misconduct.'

'Don't you think there is too much discrimination against bearded men? Even Abdul Sattar Edhi got detained at New York's JFK Airport in 2008, just for his beard. Some would argue we should be fighting against this prejudice.'

'Personally, I agree. It is sad this mistake and the widespread Islamophobia are still going on. But I am not in the business of protest and agitation. Fact is, most militants involved in the FATA insurgency are bearded and all I wish to do is ensure our rescuers have the least threatening appearance. In saying that, I do not dismiss them for a beard.'

As our conversation has touched on the subject of Abdul Sattar Edhi, I use the opportunity to explore Dr Naseer's relationship with the original guru of ambulance services.

'You know I will never say a bad word against Edhi. He is a special man, a saint, you could say.'

Dr Naseer goes on to explain how initially he wanted to help the Edhi Foundation develop by offering to educate its ambulance staff. Using the infrastructure already in place made sense. But as it would be a government initiative, Edhi was opposed. While Naseer respected Edhi's desire for independence, he knew in the end that to get the service he envisaged he would need to start afresh.

'Edhi's ambulances will always play a role in patient transport and body removal. But making paramedics out of drivers is mostly impossible.'

Dr Naseer leans back in his chair, this time asking me a question. 'Our ambulances will reach the scene in less than seven minutes,' he says, 'So tell me, what is your average response time in Sydney?'

Like any director of an ambulance service, I presume Dr Naseer would care little for my opinion that short response times actually matter in far fewer cases than people imagine. As for Rescue 1122's seven-minutes claim, internally collated statistics are highly suspicious in any country, least of all one as famed for corruption as Pakistan, where data will always support stakeholder objectives. Be that as it may, I flatter my friend by telling him our Australian figures are closer to ten minutes despite our extensive resources, which tickles his fancy, prompting him to ring the bell on his desk triumphantly and order in some coffee and sweets.

Once lunch is over Dr Naseer performs his prayers and I wait for him on the sprawling verandah overlooking the academy's parade ground where four hundred recruits are standing to attention under the beating sun. Any discomfort they may feel is undetectable, their eyes are front, faces glistening with the sweat running from under their cherry-red helmets. So straight are their backs they could have been pressed by the same iron that flattened the long-sleeve uniforms they wear. The furrow-browed parade leader, flanked by flag bearers carrying both the Pakistani and Rescue 1122 flags, marches around with rapid flicks of his lower legs. On his approach to a concrete podium, pinned with more flagpoles, he gives a series of almighty goosesteps before coming to attention with a flourish of boot stamping, as if he is trying to trample a dangerous scorpion. This reminds me of the famous gate-closing ceremony at the Wagah border with arch rival India only 40 kilometres down the road, a theatrical drill competition for army officers from both sides, cheered on by punters sitting in tiered stadium-like seating.

When I first started as an ambulance officer in 1996 we also performed a march, albeit a shoddy effort practised twice for the purpose of something to do on graduation day. Australia may be a mutual member of the British Commonwealth, but the Pakistanis have made it a national obsession to keep alive – even exaggerate – the pomp and ceremony of their former occupiers.

The contrast between this impressive battalion of paramedics and the ambulance drivers of Abdul Sattar Edhi's 115 is obvious. Edhi's stories of being a young man in the most brutal final days of the Raj are horrendous and his dislike of British rule and its legacy is deep-seated. It's unlikely he'd find the pomposity of this paramedic display as entertaining as I do. Nor would my unruly Pashtun friends in the northwest of the country who consider this Punjabi peacockery particularly irritating.

How marching has any relevance to the assistance of the sick or injured was a question put to the Ambulance Service of New South Wales by its officers more than ten years ago. Neither nurses nor doctors march around like soldiers, so why should paramedics? Without a satisfactory answer, an era of passing-out parades finally came to an end.

In Dr Naseer's opinion, however, marching is a necessity in Pakistan. 'Let me say it openly. My countrymen have a reputation for being a bit wild, a bit loose, you know, in need of some discipline. And efficiency, I believe, is directly linked to discipline.'

Though I agree with him in theory, I wonder just how different Edhi's and Naseer's staff are in terms of *actual* effectiveness on-road. After all, some of the most laid-back paramedics I've worked with in Australia are the most competent, while the neatest among them can be out of touch, socially awkward or clinically inept.

Taking me down a shady corridor of arches Dr Naseer approaches a fit, knuckle of a man with spectacles and perfectly manicured moustache. 'Let me introduce you to our head of curriculum,' he says. 'This is Dr Farhan.'

The man salutes me, waiting for his boss to finish.

'Farhan will take you for a walk through our training grounds to see what our recruits for rural Punjab are doing. My managers have been told to provide you every courtesy. If there is anything else you need, just call me.'

After apologising about his inability to spend a lazy week sipping drinks at the Country Club again, Dr Naseer disappears, trailing his entourage of assistants.

It's relatively easy in Pakistan, if dressed well and possessing a bit of regal bearing, to be treated with reverence. Attendant respect is multiplied when strolling through the rescue academy alongside Dr Farhan and his colleagues. At every turn I'm saluted and all my attempts to connect with a humble handshake instead elicit profuse apologies followed by a succession of extra salutes to reinforce the acceptable convention among these Pakistani medics.

Spread across a vast dirt training ground, four or five hundred recruits are busy at separate activity stations. As we move between them, each station springs to life like a motion-activated diorama. It's as if these hundreds of trainee rescuers and their lecturers have been patiently awaiting our arrival to show off their skills. Seems my desire for fly-on-the-wall observation has been subverted by Dr Naseer's cabaret of lifesaving, well rehearsed for official visits.

Rows of young men with military buzz cuts sit cross-legged in precise rows, looping knots under the watchful eye of a rugged old brigadier. Those mistakenly tying a granny knot instead of a reef knot are severely reprimanded, forced to perform a painful series of somersaults on the stony earth of the training ground. During my visit in 2004, discipline for paramedics was meted out in the form of fifty push-ups supervised by sergeant-majors of the Elite Police Force wielding bamboo canes. I still recall the pity I felt for one poor student struggling to complete his push-ups under my chalkboard diagram of the female reproductive system after failing to correctly identify the fallopian tubes.

An elaborate rubble-field has been constructed adjacent to the knot station and I'm surprised to see it supervised by a female. Ms Tahira Khan has almost too gentle and pretty a face to belong to a rescue trainer. As I get nearer though, I see it is crossed by two neat scars that give her a certain toughness which I imagine would be handy in the man's world she inhabits. Standing atop a mound of broken concrete from a partially collapsed building nearby, Tahira removes her silk headscarf, passing it to an assistant who gives her a pair of protective goggles and hard hat.

Once geared up, she yanks the pull-switch on the side of a jackhammer used for the extrication of people trapped under concrete. An image of my father struggling to start our family lawnmower back in Sydney springs to mind. As a child I felt such pity for him, my father, my hero, flinging up his sweaty arm over and over, cursing with frustration. When Tahira Khan fails to start the motor the first few times, a male colleague offers to pull it for her. But she orders him to back off and promptly tries again. On the fourth go the motor springs to life and she lifts up a set of 25-kilogram spreaders – the jaws-of-life – slipping its giant pincer teeth around a length of industrial steel protruding from the rubble, her face taut with concentration. As the metal groans, bends and splits in two, Tahira looks pleased.

She is a little breathless when she pulls off her mask, but manages to give me a broad smile. It's obvious to all this is more than just a rescue demonstration. Women in Pakistan are as interested in proving to the world they are making progress in gender equality as they are in fighting their menfolk to achieve it. Too often, Tahira told me later, the West assumes Pakistani women are all burqa-clad and downcast. On the flipside, few topics irritate progressive Pakistani females more than Western interpretation of the headscarf as a symbol of oppression. For many Muslim women like Tahira Khan, her insistence on wearing the hijab has become part protest at such ignorance of their right to modesty. And so, after removing her hard hat, Tahira puts her hijab back on, brushes the rock dust off her uniform and sees us to the next training station.

'Are there many ladies like you working on the ambulances here?' I ask her as we walk together.

'Unfortunately no. We encourage it, of course, but not many apply for the job in the first place. It is still early days for us, perceptions of gender roles are still a bit old fashioned.'

In Australia the first female paramedics only began work as late as the mid 1970s. Even then, female officers wore pleated skirts, carried their handbags to emergencies and were allowed to do little more than pass their male counterparts items of equipment when requested.

'In Pakistan the issue of nightshift is problem too because female staff feel very uncomfortable on duty with large group of men during evening. And as you can imagine, husbands will also worry about this situation. Still, we want to boost female numbers and will always find roles for them.'

Standing under a steel tower 105 feet tall with Rescue 1122 painted up its side, Tahira Khan advises me to ready my camera. Another female rescuer is about to abseil from the top of the tower, face first. Demonstrations like this are about entertainment value and by no means reflect the real-life application of techniques. And as anyone who has visited the country will know, patriotism is essential to any official or public display in the Punjab. So I'm hardly surprised to see the abseiling woman unfurl a Pakistani flag behind her as she hurtles down towards us. Just metres from the earth she flips over, plants her boots in the dust with a thud, unclips her ropes and salutes her audience. Impressive.

Before leaving the 'rescue from height' station, I'm rather unsettled by another officer descending with a patient lashed to his back. Normally a cage-like stretcher known as a 'Stokes litter' is used for such retrievals. My concern for the volunteer victim's welfare is not unfounded. Reaching the base of the tower, efforts are made to loosen the patient's ropes and I see he is not only barefoot and dressed in convict rags, but covered from head to toe in bruises of every vintage. As the patient limps away I notice his elbows and knees are raw with fresh abrasions, his legs spotted with blisters, his face swollen and blighted by a nasty black-eye. How is it a person would voluntarily submit themselves to such a battering? Usually, anywhere else in the world, lifelike plastic manikins are used for training and simulations and they commonly end up in horrendous shape. Could it be that in this poverty-stricken country where the have-nots are ready to perform any job, no matter how unpleasant, manikins are simply unnecessary? Is it true what I hear, that prisoners of the state and homeless men collected from the streets of Lahore are employed in this capacity? Pakistani drug companies are well known to freely exploit down-and-outs for experiments and drug trials, so why wouldn't Rescue 1122 have themselves a few living manikins?

Head-to-toe assessment of the emergency patient is an essential skill for paramedics the world over and groups of rescue medics huddle in small teams frisking one another for injuries, pretending to check their palms every now and then for blood. In Pakistan, this head-to-toe assessment is curiously known as 'axilla-to-toe', which, for the non-medical person means armpit-to-toe, and is most odd indeed considering the incidence of critical head trauma has forever outweighed that of the injured armpit.

Manning the assessment station is a thickset instructor who beckons us to wait before we go on. He pulls me close, whispering in my ear.

'In your country, sir, you do this assessment?'

'Of course,' I reply. 'But we start at the head.'

'Very good, sir. I have question, can I ask?'

'Sure.'

'Sir, do you have one special cup?'

'Cup?'

'Yes, sir, special cup for the private part of patient, for protection of that private part during axilla-to-toe assessment, so as not to brush this very sensitive private part?'

'No, we don't have a cup. We just *avoid* those parts.'

The cultural consequences of such an intimate assessment have not previously entered my mind and I'm suddenly conscious of the problems these officers will likely face in the field while carrying it out. Pertaining to unfamiliar women, it's common knowledge that Pakistani gentlemen are forbidden a mere sideways glance. Yet here, at Rescue 1122, six hundred men are about to be issued official permits to professionally feel them up. Although I've no reason to question the integrity of the service's carefully vetted recruits, it isn't surprising the last intake attracted twenty-five thousand applications.

Cardio pulmonary resuscitation (CPR) is performed en masse nearby. Fifty or so Resusci-Annes are laid out in long, precise rows with rescuers pumping up and down on each of their chests, stopping only to puff a couple of breaths into clammy, half-open mouths. No hygienic bag-valve-mask ventilation is in sight. A lack of training equipment is no doubt to blame. But how impeccable is their timing! Counting compressions aloud in Urdu at the top of his voice, another parade-ground leader struts up and down slapping on the head anyone out of sync.

'Ek! Do! Teen! Char!' and so on he yells, watching his students drip sweat onto their dolls, suffering in the 40-degree heat. Resusci-Anne is unperturbed. That plastic and rubber bust, lovingly shaped by her Norwegian inventor Asmund Laerdal and modelled from the death mask of a drowned *mademoiselle* pulled out of the Seine in 1888, lies here in this Pakistani dustbowl more than a hundred years later. Crusty beggars as living manikins for CPR practice couldn't possibly compete with the sublime allure of Annie. Genuine chest compressions would be way too painful anyway, even for the toughest hobo getting top rupee.

My tour is all a bit reminiscent of James Bond exploring Q's laboratory, even the use of both artificial and live human victims. Three men grasp a fire hose and extinguish the shell of a Volkswagen Beetle set alight for my benefit. As we pass, their eyes flick nervously in my direction, hoping to catch a look of approval. Nearby, acrid black clouds billow from a specially built smoke room. Two rescuers in breathing apparatus shout their pressure readings and charge into the darkness. After five minutes of suspense they emerge with a sooty figure I'm relieved to see is a full-sized manikin.

At the final station, the canal rescue team is engaging in synchronised star-jumping at the edge of a deep rectangular pool of murky water. Under orange buoyancy vests the size of dinner jackets, they wear swimming trunks with a 1930s look and appear more like a dance troupe rehearsing for the Mardi Gras than a serious rescue outfit.

'These men go without scuba gear and dive suits?' I ask the colonel in charge, appalled at the idea of jumping into the filthy canals of Lahore for body retrievals.

'People think they are sewers,' he replies, 'but you know, they are not so bad these days.'

Not so bad? Last time my taxi took Canal Road, the stench forced me to wind up my window and pinch my nose.

Dr Farhan interjects.

'We only employ the dedicated ones,' he says, which I take to mean 'those willing to do just about anything'. Indeed, few jobs outside the military are quite as competitive in Pakistan as Rescue 1122. An exceptionally rigorous recruitment process – including 'phobia evaluation' where applicants are placed in deep underground holes and dangled by the feet from hundred-foot towers – has been designed to ensure only the toughest and most committed are selected. Candidates as timid as I am about rappelling face-first or swallowing polluted canal water are quickly eliminated.

'Too many government jobs in Pakistan are attained through bribery and nepotism,' says Dr Farhan. 'But Rescue 1122 is different. Our leader, Dr Naseer, is a very moral man. He strongly believes in selection on merit. That is why we have rescuers even from poor families. Rescue work can only be carried out by people selected on merit. Those coming in by other means will be easily and quickly discovered.'

Joining Rescue 1122 has become, for many, a more attractive alternative to military service at a time when the Pakistan Army has close to a hundred thousand troops fighting insurgents along the country's western border and when its soldiers are expected, on a regular basis, to fire on their own countrymen. Despite opposition to extremism and the Taliban way of life, plenty of Pakistani army personnel have defected in protest at the violent and counterproductive manner in which these threats are quashed. Becoming a rescuer, on the other hand, provides an opportunity to help fellow Pakistanis without having to shoot them, offering something positive to the country while still getting a taste of that thrilling discipline.

Before we leave the training ground, I witness a parade review as forty or so rescuers stand rigidly as toy soldiers on either side of a brass band. There are six women too, helmets strapped tightly over black *hijabs*, two of them struggling to suppress the giggles. As we approach, the musicians cut loose with a flourish of cymbals, the bass drum speeds up its thumping and the clarinetist launches into an improvised swing-jazz number with an oriental twist, his cheeks puffing out like cupcakes.

From the high window of my room in the guest quarters of a newly built station just out of town, I watch two medics hose down an ambulance and restock it for nightshift. My feet are cold against the tiles but as soon as I'm conscious of this there is a knock at my door and a little man scurries in with a pair of fluffy slippers. One after the other he puts them on my feet. His name is Ajmal and from his rescue tracksuit it appears he may be a trained medic. But his assignment today is that of loyal servant to the foreigner. From the time I arrived half an hour ago, the fellow has been unable, even for a moment, to leave me unattended. With the exception of five-star hotels, few places on earth remain where a guest is so revered, where an ordinary man can be treated with such extraordinary respect.

'Anything else, sir?' asks Ajmal, eyes lowered.

'No mate, you take it easy, won't you?'

Once Ajmal has left the room I do not hear his thongs go down the corridor and suspect the man is lingering outside. I creep to the closed door and wrench it open. There he is, my private sentinel with a straight back and stern expression. He doesn't flinch at my surprise and coolly gives me a brisk salute.

'Sir, what is it I can get?'

'Nothing right now, thank you.'

'Sir, it is my duty to be all for you, sir. What about some dinner, sir? Sir wants I bring him some dinner?'

Picking up dinner would at least allow Ajmal a change of scenery from the corridor outside my room, so I nod and he races down the stairs in the way he would to a fire call. Moments later I hear his motorbike speed away up the road. It's clear Ajmal has missed the opportunity for a leisurely break when he returns less than half an hour later, breathless and soaked in sweat, carrying a paper bag. Carefully, as if handling bone china, he unwraps several pieces of cold fried chicken, a stack of sliced white bread, a tray of limp potato chips and ten sachets of tomato ketchup. Pakistani impressions of the Western diet and the sincere efforts of locals to provide their foreign guests with a slice of home is quite touching. But ever since I was served an icing-slathered birthday cake for dinner by a friend's family the charm has, for the most part, worn off. Chicken from FFK or CFK or KKF or whatever other acronym of KFC the local fry-up has chosen to use may not be nutritious, though I look pleased so as not to offend Ajmal and tell him there is nothing further. He ignores me, and stays to watch as I chow down, leaning over to refill my glass of water from a jug every time I take a sip.

In the morning I begin work at the rescue service's Central Station, so I am keen to get an early night. Dr Naseer has sent me over a green uniform, the one his rescuers wear. Ajmal has ironed and hung it up ready. Under blankets printed with giant flowers I drift off to sleep, sparing a thought as I do for poor Ajmal, loyal servant and lone sentry, keeper of a cold corridor, wide awake until dawn.

Like many travellers through rural areas of the subcontinent, I have often marvelled at the pillars of hay teetering on rickety donkey carts without considering the poor farmers risking their lives in the shadows of such loads. Not once as a medic in the outback of Australia was I sent to anyone 'trapped under a haystack' but the ambulance crew with whom I am assigned to work attend such mishaps regularly and it is to one of these we have just been dispatched.

Jaws clenched with determination, brows creased in concern, this new breed of Pakistani paramedic carries an aura of such superhuman ability they could have been lifted from the pages of a comic book. Sandwiched between two of them in the front seat of a Mercedes Sprinter, pushing through the peak-hour traffic of Lahore, I may indeed be riding shotgun with Batman and Robin or swinging through the jungle on Tarzan's ropey vines. While paramedics in many countries are taken for granted, here they are showered with adoration. Evening commuters wave from the pavement as we pass. They whistle from cars and lean out of bus windows to cheer us on. They punch the air and yell at the tops of their voices, '1122 Zindabad! Long live 1122!'

On my left sits Mohammad Azam, officer-in-charge of the Central Station close to the heart of Lahore's old city, who every so often mutters the words 'safely, safely, safely' as we edge through intersections bustling with rickshaws, donkey carts and buses coughing exhaust. Our driver Khalid scans the road ahead, his cheeks riddled with scars as severe as shrapnel wounds. Riding in the back is Pashtun paramedic Naeem Khan – to his colleges known simply as 'Khan' – a short man with a pencil-thin moustache who pokes his face through a little peephole every so often in order to gauge our progress. Whenever he does this, Azam loudly fires the same question at his star paramedic.

'Are you ready for next emergency?'

'Yes sir! I am ready!' declares Khan.

All three men – Azam, Khalid the driver and Khan – have carried on like this the entire day. If Pakistan had *Thunderbird* puppets, these would be them. How much of this camp hoo-ha I wonder is for show and how much is genuine routine? Taking oneself this seriously is an exhausting exercise and could never, surely, be sustained for as long as these men have been in the job. What ridicule would follow were I to ask my own paramedic partners back home if they are 'ready for next emergency'. You must be kidding, they would answer. We're ready for lunch, that's what we're ready for. Learn to relax, mate.

Taking us to the outskirts of the city where the buildings are thinning out to farmland we see a man waving and beckoning us to follow him. He scampers down a dirt track along a field of turned earth, forcing us to leave the sealed road. Already dented from five years' hard labour in Lahore city, the ailing Mercedes bounces in and out of gaping potholes before coming to a stop at the precipice of a lethal crater into which the dirt track has disappeared altogether.

'By foot! By foot we go!' cries Azam, leaping out and retrieving a bag of neck collars from the side door of the ambulance. Khan pulls the trolley from the back and we circumnavigate the crater, arriving at a group of villagers huddling around a man covered in dust and straw, clutching his chest, uttering groans of pain.

Khan takes immediate charge of the patient while Azam politely requests the crowd to move away and allow the man to be lifted and laid flat on the trolley, his neck stabilised with a hard collar. Every other procedure will be done en route to hospital, the best practice when it comes to trauma.

'His body crushed under haystack,' says Khan as I climb in behind him. 'I will give him a painkiller.'

We crawl back up to the main road. Despite the ambulance swaying from side to side as Khalid does his best with the potholes, Khan manages to sink an IV with nimble fingers, as quickly as the best intensive care paramedics I know. Azam passes him a bag of isotonic solution, followed by a syringe of Diclofenac Sodium for the pain. Stocks of Diclofenac, an effective non-steroidal anti-inflammatory drug also known as Voltaren, come cheap in

Pakistan nowadays since its use in the treatment of cattle was shown to be toxic to vultures feeding on carcasses. Last year the vulture population came close to extinction. Because these birds play an essential role in the maintenance of public health, their disappearance would have devastated Pakistan, and the use of Diclofenac in livestock was banned.

Opiates are just as cheap – a vial of morphine can be bought for less than a dollar by health services anywhere in the world. But Dr Naseer has avoided introducing opium-based analgesia due to the widespread abuse of narcotics in Pakistan's public hospitals. Poorly paid nurses, even doctors, have been known to steal and re-sell restricted drugs or, in moments of stress and despondency, become addicted themselves.

'Look, here,' says Khan as he performs an armpit-to-toe assessment. 'He has pneumothorax.'

It surprises me that Khan should suggest the presence of a collapsed lung given he has not yet auscultated the patient's breath sounds with a stethoscope. Sensing my scepticism, Khan takes my hand and places it over the man's left chest, pushing my fingertips into the intercostal spaces between the ribs. He looks up, watching my reaction.

'You feel?'

Sure enough, just below the surface of the skin I detect small lumps of air moving like bubble-wrap.

'Subcutaneous emphysema,' I say.

Khan looks pleased. In my time as a paramedic I've dealt with a mere handful of punctured lungs, most often satisfied with a diagnosis based on unequal and decreased breath sounds. Khan, on the other hand, encounters a pneumothorax almost weekly. Such is the level of trauma in Lahore.

At Jinnah Hospital, the city's Level 1 trauma centre named after Pakistan's founder, Mohammad Ali Jinnah, our driver mops the ambulance and Azam congratulates Khan on a job well done.

'You satisfied by treatment?' Azam asks his charge.

'Yes, sir!' Khan replies.

'You satisfied with nurses at hospital?'

A shy smile creases Khan's earnest face.

'Sir, very much, sir.'

This brief, lighthearted exchange is reassuring. Perhaps they are not such a serious bunch after all. It always takes time opening up to strangers, allowing them to see the reality, and most especially foreigners clutching notepads and film cameras and arriving with an unclear agenda, ready to document every move and every word. As if reading my mind, Mohammad Azam's chest puffs out and his face returns to that of a chiselled hero.

'Driver Khalid, Officer Khan, are you ready both for next emergency? Tell me! Tell me!'

'Yes, sir!' they reply in unison. 'We are ready!'

Sunsets viewed through heavy Pakistani smog are the most beautiful to behold. Standing on the rooftop of Lahore's Central Ambulance Station I watch the city dusted in a rich bronze light and share a cigarette with the station's security guard, his matt-black Winchester shotgun at the ready. There is something inherently contradictory about a man armed like some commando with the word 'Rescuer' embroidered on his shirt. As the paramedics of Johannesburg and Jerusalem who choose to carry a weapon would say, any defiance of the Red Cross principles is for their own survival. A dead rescuer is good for nothing and the priority of every paramedic worldwide is self-preservation. Pakistanis work in a risky environment where attacks by insurgents on government facilities have become a regular occurrence. On 15 October 2009 six people were killed and seven wounded when militants raided the Elite Police Training Centre where I gave my lectures to the first batch of paramedics in 2004. Press photos of the parade ground where men like Mohammad Azam and Naeem Khan graduated, showed bleeding and dead policemen scattered about like tin soldiers.

Memories of the grand display at the launch of Punjab's rescue service flood back. Volunteer actors playing victims that day were spreadeagled on the same burning concrete while Dr Naseer's new recruits went about demonstrating their life-saving abilities. Had the Rescue 1122 headquarters not shifted to Ferozpur Road, paramedics may well have been among the dead. As the blast I'd narrowly missed at Peshawar's district courts demonstrated, no institution, no matter how noble its cause, is immune to attack. Dr Naseer's highest profile ambulance station has been encircled by a perimeter of steel barriers painted in candy-stripe and entwined with rolls of barbed wire, a strategy to prevent car or truck bombers from getting too close to the building. It is a moderate precaution in comparison to some. After its sister establishment in Islamabad was destroyed by a gigantic blast on 9 June 2009, an impenetrable wall of shipping containers was constructed around Karachi's Pearl Continental Hotel.

Mini-parades are routinely held before each shift in the confines of the plant room. As Mohammad Azam inspects the shininess of his night crew's boots he gives a motivational speech, finishing with that regular catch-cry 'Rescue! Rescue! Rescue!' echoed in unison by his team. Glancing over to where I'm standing the man slips a bit of English into his speech and delivers it as robotically as an official script he has spent a week rehearsing.

'Our objective is to provide timely rescue and quality emergency care. Rescue from height – *enjoy it*. Jumping from height – *enjoy it*. Runnings – *enjoy it*. Push-ups – *enjoy it*. Sit-ups – *enjoy it*. Because we want to serve our nation.'

Azam's eyes glance my way as he paces about like a general about to lead his men into battle.

'Daily we do CPRs on dummies. Due to our physical abilities, we can do CPR on dummies for two hours non-stopping.'

How daunting. Unless dragged from a vat of ice, if a patient is still dead after thirty minutes one can make a pretty safe bet on the outcome. Another hour and a half of CPR would do little more than induce a cardiac arrest in the person applying it. But I keep quiet.

'We are lucky to provide sense of security to our nation. Remember, we have been given name of Green Angels because our green uniform is giving peace-ness to all.'

Some 'peace-ness' in the form of a minute's silence is observed after this in memory of four rescuers bearing the names Moosa, Shafquat, Kashuf and Idrees who were killed on 20 December 2008, when Pakistan's largest multi-storey shopping mall collapsed in a fire. Rainbow-coloured portraits of the *shaheed* – the martyrs – stare down from a wall behind the bowed heads of nightshift. Last year the service almost lost another crew of medics when they were shot at during the terrorist ambush of the Sri Lankan cricket team. Later in the night I get a tour of the roundabout where the incident took place by Omar, an ambulance driver who escorted the entourage. While taking direct machine-gun fire from three Kalashnikovs, Omar managed to whisk injured cricketers to safety driving on bare rims after all four tyres of the ambulance were shot out. Bullet holes indicated thirty-five rounds had penetrated the ambulance without hitting anyone.

Immediately following this incident, Dr Rizwan Naseer seriously considered the acquisition of bulletproof ambulances until realising the cost. Unfortunately, wealthy African dictators and Catholic Popes have pushed up the price of such vehicles beyond the budget of Pakistani ambulance services.

Needless to say, Azam and his rescuers reveal little fear of anything at all and cling instead to practical action plans and protocols. Sitting among his charges at 11 pm waiting for a call,

I ask Azam how, in the event of another attack, rescuers plan on saving themselves. He answers without a moment's hesitation.

'Sah, with crawlings, sah.'

At first I don't quite get it. 'Crawlings?' I ask.

'Yes sah, crawling techniques.'

'I see.'

'Sah, we crawl beside earth, with help of knees, with foots, with arms. Sah, you will see demonstration of crawlings, let us show you.'

Promptly Azam turns to one of his men, clicks his fingers and barks, 'Please! Demonstrate!' An earnest young man with a neat haircut reacts immediately and jumps onto the tiles of Azam's office, scooting along face down like a worm on amphetamines. How it is possible for a human being to move this fast while prone is beyond me and I give a hearty clap once the man has disappeared out the door.

'His name is Mohammad Naveed,' says Azam. 'You know, sah, he is our specialist cobra catcher.'

'You have a specialist cobra catcher?' I ask, thinking it quite a handy thing the man can slither as quickly as he does.

'Sah, our good service has specialist cobra catcher but he has also caught one rabbit cat.'

'Rabbit cat?'

'Rabbit cat.'

'What kind of an animal is a rabbit cat?' I ask, perplexed. 'A cat with large ears?'

'No, no, sah. Ra-bid cat, sah.'

'Oh, a cat with rabies.'

'Sah. And most seriously, sah,' Azam says with a furrowed brow. 'This city has a big aunt-eater problem.'

Aunt-eaters would hardly be considered a nuisance by plenty of people back home, not to mention mother-in-law-eaters. Though I'm firmly assured about the surprising viciousness of

Pakistani anteaters, I remain unconvinced about the threat of such a slow-moving creature, feeding as it does on tiny insects we humans unwittingly crush underfoot each day. From his body language Mohammad Naveed gives me the impression he would rather drop the subject. Understandably, a rescuer of anteaters is far less glamorous or romantic a title than one belonging to a cobra catcher.

The dangers of ambulance work are many and varied and another medic, Hassan Hameed, rolls up his sleeve to show me a scar he acquired from being stabbed by a mentally ill patient. How this could have happened I don't know, as the rescuers are fully trained in judo, practising regularly on foam mats kept at the academy. Back in Sydney, I tell him, we do not have the benefit of martial arts to protect ourselves from agitated patients. Our biggest threat comes from the violent drunk, and when I mention this, the men are desperate to hear more. It's not unusual, I tell them, for every ambulance in the city of Sydney on Friday and Saturday nights to attend more than ten intoxicated patients consecutively. My Pakistani friends shake their heads in amazement. In his five years as a medic, Hassan has not attended a single drunk. Alcohol is *haram* – forbidden in Islam – and officially banned in Pakistan. Although many people do drink in secret here, they would rather die from whiskey poisoning than end up legless in the back of an ambulance.

Via a moped accident on a suburban street, I'm dropped back at the guest quarters where I find Ajmal standing to attention in exactly the same spot I left him in that morning. Predictably, as I go to shake his hand, he avoids my palm and salutes instead. Too tired to argue about the joys of informality I let out a sigh and collapse into bed.

During the night I'm woken now and then by distant echoes of ambulances heading out on emergencies, stretchers being hosed down, doors slamming, muffled voices in tall corridors. Occasionally as vehicles zoom off they briefly leave a flash of blue beacon light against my curtains. Fifteen years of compulsory nightshift has been enough for me and, if given a choice, few paramedics I know would volunteer for them. At the same time, however, I've always felt a tinge of disappointment about missing out on the conflict, agony and madness of the night and the stories it forever offers up.

The crowded alleys of Lahore's Old City are cluttered with every obstruction imaginable. Our ambulance negotiates mule wagons loaded with trembling towers of wooden crates, ice-cream carts and balloon-sellers crying out for customers, throngs of women gazing at embroidered fabrics, grubby-faced men carrying car parts and satellite dishes and clusters of long iron rods. Animals and children dart out from between the flowing traditional robes of elders as they spill from the arches of a small mosque, reminding our driver just how dangerous it would be driving through here too fast. But his eyes are agile, scanning left and right as our siren clears the way.

Our 'waver' is difficult to identify among the other friendly waving folk. The call is to a cardiac arrest and we have already passed the service's advertised seven-minute response time pledge so we sit stationary at the given location with the siren on, hoping to draw out the caller.

Less than thirty seconds later, Azam, Khan, the driver and I are dashing through a three-foot wide passage between buildings in hot pursuit of a breathless adolescent who is leading us to the victim. Pushing the stretcher ahead of him, the driver does his best to keep up with the rest of us. The metal frame and little wheels of the trolley clatter noisily over the cobbles, only just avoiding people stepping out from doorways on hearing the commotion.

Left then right, then right again we go until we lose our guide who, due to his state of anxiety, has run much faster. We use the moment to catch our breath before he re-emerges and leads us through a half-open door into the courtyard of a family home. It's then I realise, as we approach an old man supine and motionless on a rope bed, that we've arrived without a defibrillator. All we have to rely on is old-fashioned CPR and I assume that the oxygen kit Khan has slung over his shoulder has all the necessary equipment for bag/mask ventilation. It does, and yet, to my horror, Khan puts it aside and whips out a neatly folded hanky from his pocket. He shakes it open with a flourish and lays it delicately over the old man's face before leaning down to apply mouth-to-mouth resuscitation through it.

I'm stunned. Never have I, or any paramedic I've heard of, directly performed mouth-to-mouth on a patient at work. Standard practice involves placing a mask over the patient's face and squeezing a balloon of oxygen attached to it. For us respiratory and cardiac arrests are commonplace. Putting ourselves at constant risk from communicable diseases by doing mouth-to-mouth is unthinkable.

'Ek, do, teen, char!' Azam is over the old man's chest doing compressions and the knots of the rope bed creak like a tethered ship in a storm. Huddled in a corner of the room a group of women whimper quietly, their eyes glistening with tears behind their veils. Meanwhile, the old man's sons pace about wringing their hands, watching our every move.

To remain a mere observer in a case like this is impossible. Furthermore, my Pakistani counterparts have made it clear I am welcome to share my knowledge with them.

'Azam, your driver, maybe he could run and bring the defibrillator from the ambulance?'

'Sah, of course, sah,' replies Azam between chest compressions, before ordering our driver back to the car.

While we wait for his return, I assemble the bag–mask. Khan has had some difficulty in performing effective head tilt with the patient lying on the rope bed and the old man has regurgitated into his beard. Khan's little brown handkerchief is soaked through with vomit. Seeing a bag–mask combination come his way, the relieved Pashtun medic folds up his hanky, slipping it back into his pocket ready for the next job.

On questioning the family more thoroughly, it becomes apparent the old man has been 'down' longer than we first realised. His pupils, when I check them, are fixed and dilated and the man's body is not particularly warm to touch. Once the defibrillator arrives it gives no commands for a shock either, strongly suggesting asystole – a flatline, a heart in complete standstill. Perhaps I've had a bad run, but asystoles I've treated have usually been refractory and even with intravenous adrenalin will merely change to a rhythm for the duration of the drug's effect. Adrenalin is not at hand, which kind of defeats the point of wasting time carting the old man to hospital while performing CPR en route, for the very same outcome.

Azam takes the sons aside and delivers the news; that we tried our best but nothing more can be done and it must surely be the old man's time to meet his maker. God is great, *Allahu Akbar*, I hear him say. Cries go up from the women and one of them hits her head with her hands over and over again. Without the language to comfort the family, I can do little else but quietly gather our gear. Grieving is natural and important and not something a paramedic is able to 'fix' anyway, even back home.

Khan binds the old man's wrists and ankles together and wraps a folded triangular bandage under his chin and around his head and does this so quickly I can tell he has already done it hundreds of times before. As there is commonly a viewing at Islamic burials, it's easier to close the jaw and neaten a body's limbs before rigor mortis sets in.

Pulling away past the leaning ramparts of the Old City, I cannot resist asking Naeem Khan about the kiss of life he was so quick and willing to perform on a complete stranger.

'Did you rinse your mouth?' I ask him.

'Sir, I will be later rinsing.'

'How many times have you given strangers mouth-to-mouth resuscitation?'

'Sir, I do not count the times. But I am guessing more than one hundred.'

'With use of that handkerchief only?'

'Sir, yes sir, the hanky is a trusty friend.'

'What do your teachers say about this?'

'Our managers put question to us, how is it possible we can teach mouth-to-mouth to the public if not willing to practice it ourselves? This is matter of honour for us in Rescue 1122. If my commitment to patient is true and from the heart, then I will do anything, am I right?' Here, noble principles win over safe clinical practice once again.

Later, when I ask Dr Farhan about the matter, he denies encouraging mouth-to-mouth and blames a lack of bag–mask equipment rather than the noble self-sacrifice of his rescuers. Naeem Khan and his colleagues, on the other hand, make it very clear their attitude to mouth-to-mouth is pure devotion. It occurs to me that Abdul Sattar Edhi's refusal to wear gloves while collecting body parts is no different. Responding with disgust – or 'cringing' as Edhi would say – is more of an enemy to a Pakistani rescuer than any illness or disease acquired through cross-infection.

While ambulance services in the West go to great lengths in reminding employees about their responsibilities to uphold organisational values, these Pakistani rescuers need nothing of the sort. In sharp contrast to the shameful corruption of the elite who have brought their country to near collapse on more than one occasion, these men and women live an extreme code of ethics. As we keep seeing on the evening news, all over Pakistan common people are ready to fight and die for what they believe in, whether it is patriotism or religion or freedom or all of these things combined. For Rescue 1122 it is first and foremost the saving of lives. I have even heard Azam refer to this as a form of 'jihad' – a noble struggle. Fear of injury or disease in the course of a struggle is considered shameful, as the suffering of jihad is important in coming nearer to Allah. And should one go so far as to die for a just cause, well, one is transformed into a martyr. What then do Naeem Khan and his colleagues have to fear from a spot of herpes simplex after mouth-to-mouth?

Conversing openly with burly Pakistani firemen and rescuers on matters of philosophy and metaphysics is most refreshing. Adult males are not the least bit shy about discussing religious faith or their admiration of nature or the poetry of Sufis. It's a welcome change from the subjects of football and women I regularly engage in back home. Even the daily text messages Mohammad Azam sends me read as if from a book of motivational quotes. 'No man can buy back his past, so live each day like the last' and just this morning, 'If your thoughts are the tree, your actions are the fruit, so what kind of fruit do you bear?'

Next door is a control room for all of Lahore, where telephones ring ceaselessly day and night. A row of men on swivel chairs mechanically lift receivers and put them down again, sometimes once every two or three seconds. Most calls do not necessitate dispatch of a vehicle and are entered into the database under a long list of categories like 'gossip calls' or 'fake calls' or 'annoying kid calls'. The operators' arduous jobs are thankfully made easier by a round-the-clock masseur with the name of Rodney, the spelling of which I assume to be more like Rahdini. Whatever the case, we find him seated on a high chair with his tight sleeves wrapped around Popeye arms, like a circus strongman. Azam introduces us and Rodney offers me the end of a raw carrot stick he's been gnawing on, which I politely decline.

'My men are very obedient,' Azam says earnestly. 'Sir, let the good Rodney ease your shoulders with his talent.'

He nods to Rodney and once the man gets going he certainly has the touch. Dispatchers in Western nations could only dream about having a Rodney around.

Unfortunately my massage is interrupted by the call to a motor vehicle accident in which a three-wheeled auto-rickshaw has gone into a city fountain.

Extricating someone from the back of a rickshaw while immobilising their spine is a challenge even without being doused in water. Making matters worse is a crowd of onlookers who have surrounded the scene with as much regard for personal space at an accident scene as they have on a common bus. It's been this way at every motor crash our ambulance has attended. As my irritation mounts I'm ready to elbow one dim-witted gloater out of the way when Azam takes command and orders everyone to retreat with a calm and generous smile.

'What did you say?' I asked.

'Sah, I told them Allah will reward their concern for fellow man, but even a Good Samaritan needs to go home.'

I'm certain then I have never met a gentleman as charming as Mohammad Azam and think how right Dr Naseer was in choosing him to head his Central Station. 'Stand back!' has long been the catch-cry of medics in Sydney who ought perhaps to be worried about their task rather than organising nosy onlookers. But in Pakistan these crowds can suck every last vestige of oxygen from an accident scene. Ordering them back is pure necessity, and doing this without causing a riot is a talent Mohammad Azam has clearly perfected.

He elaborates further on the rubbernecks while our driver cleans up.

'My worry is for them; it is dangerous. They just stand there in middle of road without thought. Some I have seen hit by other vehicles, seriously injured. People have more time here to stop and look and get in way of us. There is lack of education.' Also, I suggest to him, Western society is more private. People keep to themselves and avoid being rude or interfering or appearing too nosy. But in a country of close-knit communities and extended families, where poverty forces people to live side by side and on top of one another, life and death become very public.

At our next motorcycle accident, Khan and the driver roll a groaning middle-aged patient onto a spine board and apply a neck collar. Twenty cars, mopeds and bicycles assemble behind the ambulance with engines idling, fingers pointing and necks craning. Avoiding a crowd is as simple as a fast load and the medics whisk him as quickly as they can to the waiting ambulance.

'Does he have neck pain?' I ask Khan as we pull out.

'No, sir, we are having some precaution.'

Dr Farhan was very clear on this point when I raised it on my tour of the new academy. Every patient involved in a crash gets a neck collar if they are willing because the service is not yet confident its medics can definitively rule out spinal injuries. Precautionary neck collars are common practice worldwide, but usually only those with pain or deficits or a decreased consciousness get one. Perhaps those involved in a serious high-speed collision also qualify as the probability of injury is greater, even without detectable symptoms and signs, and especially if intoxicated or suffering some other distracting injury. Rescue 1122 medics are 'technicians' rather than 'clinicians', which must be the wisest approach when training large numbers of people to perform a job that has not previously existed, and for which there are few experienced mentors. In a way I envy these medics – because there is less pressure on them to make precise clinical judgments, their treatments err heavily on the side of caution.

Hospital staff in Lahore are not so pleased about this constant stream of supine patients wheeled in with neck collars in place. Before Rescue 1122 began, the same patients would arrive by rickshaw and sit in the waiting room. Now they all come in the back door, straight onto a bed. Road traffic accidents represent about 80 per cent of the work the rescue service performs, and hospitals struggle to keep up with the influx. Compared to most Western nations they do remarkably well for the number of casualties received. Whenever our team arrives at an Accident and Emergency (A&E) room there is a bed waiting and we offload without delay. It helps that emergency beds are pushed together so closely they are almost touching. In Sydney three of these beds could fit into a cubicle designed for one. In Pakistan, where there's a greater tolerance for lack of personal space, a patient will rarely wait for a hospital bed. Instead, they'll end up lying near enough to the next injured man to satiate their curiosity about his condition without ruining their eyesight.

For a week or more I'm with Mohammad Azam and Naeem Khan and the driver. Every day we work non-stop. Their turnarounds are lightning fast and their energy unrelenting. This is quite remarkable considering they only get four days off each month.

One morning when I arrive at work I'm asked to look over an 'improvement list' handed to me by a manager whose uniform I suspect has been altered by a tailor for an extra tight fit. Categories on the list focus on behaviour, appearance and discipline of staff with very little about their state of morale or, for that matter, clinical competence. A few short stints as Acting Station Officer in New South Wales has hardly prepared me for making recommendations to Pakistani ambulance managers, but I'm grilled on strategies to ensure a professional workforce and the manager insists I join him and senior executives at the Rescue Academy for lunch.

Just then, Mohammad Azam arrives with a certain look of determination.

'Sah,' he says urgently, 'grains.'

Motioning for me to hold out my palm he drops a scattering of corn kernels and channa peas into it. His eyes twinkle under that dark and serious brow and I know that in just a week we've become good friends. Only the night before I'd received a text message on my mobile phone from him that read, 'Promises and friends are like snowballs. Easy to make, but difficult to keep.' I replied that I hoped our friendship would never melt.

Upstairs we sit with Khan and the day shift that has not yet been dispatched and we all sip Lipton Yellow Label tea from dainty old-lady teacups.

'How many dry fruit you experience in this country?' enquires one medic while distributing raisin-like morsels among his colleagues from a little paper envelope.

'Not many,' I reply.

'Well sir, *inshallah*, we will help you experience many dry fruit.' And there is a mumble of agreement all round.

Later, at the Rescue 1122 headquarters, I sit at a table wide enough for a royal banquet and listen to the arguments of the service's top brass, watching them scoop handfuls of curry with hot *roti* into their mouths. Dr Naseer is unable to join us due to a meeting at Jinnah Hospital. Although I understand much less of the discussions in Urdu than I should, I soon become suspicious something sinister or subversive is being plotted. Voices hush every time the door is answered or footsteps pass outside and the body language all round is decidedly cagey. I tell myself it won't be long and the mystery will be revealed, but my frustration at not knowing begins to mount unbearably. I single out a female manager and ask her what is going on. Smiling dismissively she says, 'Top secret, sir, I'm sorry.'

Outside in a deserted quadrangle, four LandCruisers wait with engines running while the executive team deliberates about who will be travelling in which car. The sun is burning and a man hands out Motorola radios to the group who fix them on their belts.

How the men relish this revival of their good old army days! Those anti-India combat exercises must have been terrific fun and even Dr Farhan, a former Pakistan Air Force doctor, is overcome with boyish excitement.

'If you really want to come with us we have to clear you with the agencies,' he says to me.

Given my ties to Pashtuns supporting the insurgency in FATA, I'm hoping the Inter-Services Intelligence doesn't vet me too closely. A radio call comes through soon after with the go-ahead. What exactly this clearance is for remains undisclosed. But motoring in convoy through the afternoon traffic of Lahore, squeezed in with cigarette-puffing rescue managers, I find the suspense exhilarating.

Arriving in the city the LandCruisers are parked about half a block away from one of the tallest buildings in the financial district of Lahore. It's a concrete monolith built around 1970. The rest of the way we travel on foot to avoid any unwanted attention that might expose the secret. Once our party reaches the shadow of the high-rise we huddle in a triangular car park opposite the building and one of the managers, with his trouser bottoms tucked into heavy boots, distributes small walnut-sized chunks of a white substance he calls *sangara*; everyone bites down or nibbles on it and only I hesitate to ask him what it is. There's some humorous banter among the group and chuckling all round before the man answers with a wink, '*Sangara* is special Pakistani herbal Viagra, it gives good energy for our mission.'

This is quite a shame because it tastes horrible and I spit it out surreptitiously behind a row of motorbikes.

After some deliberation, the men cross the road and stand behind a shoulder-high concrete wall over which they discreetly peer to scrutinise the main entrance busy with accountants and stockbrokers going about their day. I still have no idea what all the stealth is about.

Dr Farhan makes a radio call and soon after a bus packed with young men arrives at the front of the building. Quietly, about fifty of them, wearing torn T-shirts and shredded tracksuit pants, file out and up the front steps. One of them carries a big bucket stained with a murky red substance while another two lug a crate between them. Why they have not been stopped by the building security I cannot say, though I suspect they've been tipped off by the 'agencies'.

There is no more hiding now. Behind the parked bus a flatbed truck pulls up, heaped high with sticks and planks, cardboard, old tyres and other junk. These items are rapidly unloaded and dragged to the base of the building, not far from the steps leading through revolving doors to the foyer. They are then piled into a tower of scrap.

Suddenly – with a flashback to the passing-out parade of rescue students in 2004 – it dawns on me what is taking place and, more alarmingly, how it is being orchestrated.

This is a major incident exercise.

BOOM! BOOM! BOOM! Three deafening explosions emit from somewhere deep inside the building. My ears are ringing. When I look at Dr Farhan incredulously, he says, 'Fireworks, in the basement …' without blinking.

He must be joking.

Why would they *simulate* a bomb blast in a city already beset by *genuine* bomb blasts? A city where everyone is paranoid and wondering when and where the next suicide bomber will strike? It's as shocking to me as it is to the office workers who begin hurriedly exiting the building, clutching their briefcases and looking back with frightened faces.

Testing the capabilities of emergency services with a disaster exercise is a common and judicious practice worldwide. In this case, however, Rescue 1122 managers have arranged it under a code of silence. Neither the ambulance and fire crews on duty, nor the public in the street or the innocent civilians working peacefully in their offices just moments ago believe this is anything but a real event. Never could such a thing be arranged elsewhere in the world without forewarning the community and rescue staff. Imagine the uproar! Emergency services would be instantly accused of menacing the population.

Public panic and psychological trauma aside, the logic of maintaining secrecy is clear. Many paramedics have reservations about major incident exercises back home for the very *lack* of surprise involved. Managers simply call in extra staff on overtime rates and have a response strategy preplanned. Wouldn't a true test of emergency services capabilities instead catch everyone unawares, create genuine pandemonium and put real pressure on normal day crews to manage an extraordinary moment? This is precisely what I'm witnessing in Lahore – an emergency service playing a double game, as both the terrorist and the rescuer.

Metres away from me, the entertainment escalates as Dr Farhan's assistant produces a jerrycan of petrol and shakes it out over the pyramid of junk. Someone calls for a match and a torch is lit nearby and handed over. Before the heap can be ignited, however, a small rotund man wearing the creased grey *shalwar kameez* of a building janitor flaps his arms and shouts, and attempting as best he can to crash-tackle the torchbearer. His duty is to protect the office block with his life and this, it seems, is finally his moment to shine after decades of pretty much nothing happening at all. By his rage and determination I can see there is no way this little man will permit a bunch of cowboys to explode things in the basement, create panic among the office workers and set a bonfire on the front steps, no matter who they are.

But the janitor is overpowered by Rescue 1122 managers who hold him back while the stack is lit.

Whoosh! Up it goes.

Everyone backs away and the janitor looks devastated. He retreats into the building as acrid black smoke from burning rubber rises thick and fast. Birds lift from the third-floor balcony and flap away in alarm. The few office workers remaining on the top floors poke their heads out as smoke passes their windows. Below them a vast audience has formed on the street to watch the spectacle. One of the managers carrying a clipboard announces he is putting through the emergency call with his mobile phone – 1122 – and simultaneously starts a stopwatch.

A blood-curdling scream erupts from the main foyer and this is followed by other shouts and wails of shock and pain. Through the revolving doors come the victims of the blast, stumbling out like extras in a zombie movie. I see they are the young men from the bus who walked in not twenty minutes ago, probably rescue students from the academy. They appear terrifying in this gross moulage, moaning and pleading for help, splattered from head-to-toe with goat's blood. Some have prosthetic wounds strapped on with string while others wear the protruding rubber bones of compound fractures. There are open lacerations and even one gaping, eviscerated abdomen with bulging intestines of latex. Down the front steps they tumble, throwing themselves on the ground, shrieking and rolling in misery, smearing gore across the granite. Raised on a diet of B-grade Indian films from the 1980s, these men have pure melodrama pumping through their veins. So desperate have they been for an outlet, they play their parts with the exuberance of pent-up movie stars.

Less than a few minutes have gone by and we hear a siren. Around the corner comes a Rescue 1122 fire truck followed by the first ambulance. Dr Farhan and his team look chuffed at the quick response. But before the firemen have a chance to reach the bonfire, we are startled to see the building janitor reappear, huffing and puffing and frantically pulling the foyer fire hose behind him, hoping it will make the distance. Luckily for him it does and there's enough pressure in it to land an arc of water in the centre of the blaze. By the time the firemen have their hoses ready and water flowing there is little more than steaming embers remaining. The old janitor has stolen their moment and, although they curse him, in a real terror attack he'd be getting a hero citation and he'd deserve it, too.

Mohammad Azam arrives with his team then and gives me a nod of acknowledgement as the panic-stricken 'victims' clutch his ankles, pleading for help. Three other ambulances pull up in convoy as well and I wonder for a second who is looking after the rest of the city.

Meanwhile, the triaging of victims is hampered by some actors who have been instructed to interfere aggressively with rescuer efforts. As one limp patient is carted off, another wounded man starts yelling that he is the victim's brother and theatrically flings himself on top of the patient causing the stretcher-bearers to collapse in a heap. All the while, a casualty nearby with a large and indistinguishable foreign body protruding from his chest is – despite his horrific impalement – screaming incessantly with both lungs.

'The basement!' cries Azam in English for my benefit and waves his ambulance team to follow. I'm close behind them, dodging the remaining office workers fleeing the building. We descend the fire stairs two at a time and reach the basement where the explosion occurred. Here the pandemonium is equal to the chaos outside, with the added problem of total darkness. Calls for help are all around, hands tripping us up as we move among the bodies. Another team further inside swings a torch from side to side, flashing on a blood-drenched face before illuminating a curled-up 'corpse' in the corner. What a relief to see a dead one lying there nice and quiet, I think to myself. After all, how many bomb blasts have killed just one man while turning fifty others into vicious, uncooperative pests?

When Azam flicks on his own torch we see we are standing in a wide pool of blood; I remember the bucket of red liquid the men had carried into the building. Piled against a far wall blackened to the ceiling with soot are the remains of the fireworks – ash heaps, burnt cardboard, shredded casings – they must have ignited the equivalent of a New Year's Eve display.

Ambulance teams sort through patients and identify the seriously wounded. They lash them to stretchers for removal. A number of the troublemakers appear to have followed us into the basement and loom out of the dark clutching at rescuers trying to lift the injured from the bloodbath. Standing in the light of the stairwell I catch sight of the master and commander, Dr Rizwan Naseer, wearing a neat suit and tie, inspecting the proceedings. Seeing me, he smiles and his smile is that of a mischievous schoolboy. I give him a quick thumbs-up letting him know I, too, am entertained.

Later that evening when I meet Dr Naseer in his office for tea, he tells me the Home Department has registered a protest with Rescue 1122 about today's exercise and the widespread anxiety it caused in the financial district.

'Of course I'm used to tussles like this and always happy to wear a controversy. Our objective is to test our system so that we can be the best possible service in case of a real attack. Responding to a blast is like a ballet concert. How can the audience expect a good performance if we don't first rehearse it?'

Rizwan Naseer is more worried about his impending trip to Peshawar. First thing tomorrow morning he is booked on a flight and has an urgent meeting with the Chief Minister of Khyber Pakhtunkhwa. Bringing his pre-hospital care to cities on the frontier was always on the cards. But suicide bombings in Peshawar and surrounding towns are occurring at a rate of one a week. Telling Dr Naseer about my own close shave with a suicide attacker makes him nervously shift in his chair.

'Taliban, or whoever, are watching the airport, you know. I confess I'm having second thoughts about going.'

'Are you getting picked up?'

'Yes, police cavalcade.'

'Risky business,' I tell him. Police and army vehicles escorting government officials like Dr Naseer are prime targets.

'Maybe you can lend me your *shalwar kameez*?' he jokes. 'And I will go to Peshawar by rickshaw.'

Black crows cry out for scraps as they circle ominously in the early haze. It's my last morning with Mohammad Azam, Naeem Khan and many other friends I've made at the Central Station. They huddle around me now with arms draped over each other, asking question after question, interrogating me like a mob of three-year-olds. It's understandable. These men started their profession from scratch, tailor-making protocols to suit the Pakistani environment and creating an organisational culture previously undefined. As they interrogate me about how we extricate patients from crashed cars and what medication we give to asthmatics in extremis, I consider this as much a sharing of knowledge as it is a confidence boost for these medics to know they have, for the past five years, been doing it right.

How unaffected by the ills of ambulance work these men appear, how impossibly energetic and upbeat. For weeks I've been vigilant for signs of cynicism, that inevitable disease of the emergency worker, both protective and destructive in equal measure. But here there is none of it – not a hint. Perhaps the concept is completely foreign to these medics since they *are* the home of pre-hospital care in Pakistan. Could it be true they have never engaged in ironic conversation or that universal ambulance humour, black and dry? Without an 'old guard' to guide them, navigating a new terrain must have been tricky. Yet the advantage has been a complete absence of pre-existing organisational culture, where cynicism may have thrived and been passed down to subsequent generations. No miserable unshaven medics burned out by decades of trauma awaited them that first day. Instead, they have worked in the best way they could, knowing no better than to be cheerful and brazenly keen.

Cynicism among paramedics in Australia is so entrenched that Pip James, a former lecturer at the ambulance education centre in Sydney, used to insist her students write themselves a letter immediately after employment. This letter would outline the students' motives for joining the job, the way they perceived the profession and a description of the paramedics they hoped to become. The letters were then sealed and only opened again once they had returned to the school after a year on the road. As expected, the students squirmed horribly when reading their earlier sentiments. But many also learnt how insidiously tainted they had become.

It's easier to avoid cynicism, however, when patients present with genuine and pressing needs, when the service is not abused. Ambulance workers in the West generally agree that the level of disgruntlement in their job is directly proportional to the number of time-wasters they attend. When customers call for a lift to the shops, for a drink of water, for a blanket when cold, it's no surprise. If customers reserved calling ambulances for serious injuries and acute illnesses only, frustration and cynicism among paramedics would probably decline accordingly.

Another significant contributor, I'm convinced, is the actual culture of the society itself. Australia, for example, is a land of relaxed and carefree people where it has always been rather uncool to appear too eager or earnest about anything. Luckily, a little *laissez-faire* goes a long way to shield paramedics from ridicule. While Azam buoys his crew by calling them 'green angels', seasoned medics in Australia typically describe their work as 'just a job, mate'. I have always pitied the younger recruits who declare that their inspiration to enter the profession has come from hospital dramas on television. With unabashed zeal they attempt to emulate their fictional heroes, quite unaware just how comical they appear to those who have seen it all before. Sooner than later, the monotonous or truly difficult and less than glamorous nature of the work will take its toll.

With Rescue 1122, Dr Rizwan Naseer's dream could have had no better milieu in which to flourish. Thousands of fit men and many women in Pakistan are desperate for decent jobs, especially in public service. But the most significant motivator is a potent nationalistic altruism among Pakistani youth in every province. As the nation is barraged by earthquakes, floods and waves of bombings, the youth have a country to save and are desperate to repair its image on the world stage.

My wife Kass has made it her habit to tease me by describing my profession as 'the force'. For the medics of Rescue 1122 it couldn't be a more fitting title. Ex-military trainers relish exploiting the patriotism of medics who leave the academy, likening them to soldiers ready for war, a war in this case against morbidity and mortality, armed with syringes and drips, splints and oxygen. And like soldiers, they are ready to die for their nation. Indeed, the personal sacrifices made for the saving of lives are extreme. While mouth-to-mouth is probably the best example of this, Mohammad Azam also claims he has never once, in five years, stopped the ambulance to buy water. Hearing this, Naeem Khan admits that he, too, rarely drinks water on shift, nor will he take lunch out of respect for his patients. Wouldn't it be shameful, he asks me, having a full stomach while treating a patient with an empty one?

From my experience, a hungry paramedic is the worst kind one can get. Still, I have no interest in dousing the extraordinary commitment these men possess. As it was with Dr Shiraz Afridi in Peshawar, I see the footprint of Abdul Sattar Edhi's philosophies imprinted on these men, and I ask them about him.

'Without *maulana* Edhi,' says Naeem Khan, 'no one in Pakistan would understand what is ambulance. When I was child, I look to this man and want to follow him.'

Azam agrees. 'Sah, Dr Naseer is our father, and Edhi is our forefather. We have taken shape because of both.'

One of the rescuers climbs onto Azam's desk and lies supine, blinking at the ceiling. 'Please,' says Azam, 'show your last tips, any tips, best tips. Sah, this is our final chance.'

I'm tempted, for a bit of fun, to ask Naeem Khan for his hanky. Instead, I get him to bring the resuscitation kit from the ambulance to show them some bag–mask ventilation. Far greater than anything I can teach them, though, is what they have taught me. In less than a month, my lust for the job has been rejuvenated by their insatiable energy and passion to help the suffering.

Waiting for my lift to the airport, my mobile phone rings and it's the controller of the station where I stayed.

'Sir, your cricket helmet has arrived.'

'Cricket helmet?'

'From Chief of Sialkot District, sir.'

Then I remember the little man, Syed Kama Abid, and his promise to send me a gift of two soccer balls from Pakistan's famous city of sporting gear manufacturers. How *two* soccer balls have become *one* cricket helmet I'm not too sure, but I guess it has to do with my Australian nationality and the assumption it makes me an automatic cricket fanatic. In truth, I have no patience at all for the game despite constantly being told by Indians and Pakistanis how much I look like former captain Ricky Ponting.

'Give the helmet to Mohammad Azam,' I tell him.

Only after I hang up do I recall Azam's preference for badminton over cricket – just a few days earlier he lamented the closure of his favourite badminton court. Still, it's the thought that counts and I know he will value the cricket helmet forever as a symbol of our friendship.

As I'm about to board my plane at the Allama Iqbal Airport, I get a typically sentimental text message from Azam. But I have no cynicism left, at least for now, so I read it as poetry, the most beautiful send-off I could hope for:

> We r tigers of town & cities, we r riders of the days & nights, bravery is our garment, boldness is our identity. Struggle against emergency & disaster is our mission. We DO NOT afraid of death, we DO NOT loss heart in hardships, we DO NOT accept defeat. We have NO FEAR. We are strong shelter for peoples. We get HARD training to fight EASY. We give our blood to rescue nation bcz life is a game of CHANCE. We r proud to be the POLITE HELPFUL PASSIONATE LIONS of PAKISTAN. EMERGENCY SERVICE RESCUE 1122. Zindabad! We are proud to be RESCUER. Have a good flight my dear. Your best friend FOREVER, Mohammad Azam.

THE NAKED PARAMEDIC

Iceland

Huddled alone in a lofty bedroom in the Reykjavik Fire Brigade headquarters with the door locked, I contemplate all that I have learnt about nudity and my own hypocrisy on the subject. I'm no prude, but I've never liked undressing in front of strangers. It makes me uncomfortable.

Paramedics see hundreds of people in various states of undress. My work has shown me that few ordinary people are attractive without their clothes on, and I'm an ordinary man with an ordinary body. But why am I thinking about this in Iceland? A freezing volcanic island just south of the North Pole was the least likely place to advocate nudity. Yet here I am, a pathetic little coward, hiding from the 5 pm sauna.

There are plenty of places to hide at the Slökkvilið Höfuð-borgarsvæðisins – the Fire Department of Reykjavik Capital Area District. The building covers an entire block and is a legacy to the country's wealth before the *kreppa*, the economic crisis of 2008. Over a spacious plant room where late-model fire engines and ambulances are parked side by side, an entire floor of the building is dedicated to the comfort of emergency crews. Three separate lounge areas are furnished with the finest recliners, two kitchens, a library, a study, a computer room and cable television sets with a hundred channels. Rows of private luxury bedrooms brightly lit through tall windows lead off the main corridor and give the appearance of a five-star hotel. With only a handful of men on each shift the place feels empty even when everybody's in, almost like a giant abandoned space station.

So much for my expectation of dog-sled ambulances dispatched from igloos. Before the *kreppa*, Iceland enjoyed the highest standard of living in the world. Most people still own the Chevrolet, Dodge or LandCruiser they bought in this golden period, trucks with monster wheels for traversing glaciers in comfort. Iceland's love of everything big and luxurious is ample evidence of America's legacy. While Iceland may soon be part of the European Union, Reykjavik is all shopping malls and burger joints and people who speak English with Pennsylvanian accents. There is no doubt the cumulative effect of American television has affected Iceland's own culture, as it has throughout the modern world. But when it comes to the ambulance service of Iceland, America can be justifiably credited with helping revolutionise emergency medical services and saving lives.

Down the corridor I hear a voice, only for a moment, calling a name, maybe mine. Yesterday I found refuge in the disabled toilet wondering just how many disabled paramedics it takes to warrant such a thing. On the dot of 5 pm I could hear men checking every bedroom. Deputy Fire Chief Birgir Finnsson had obviously sent out a search party to find me. They know by now, all of them, about my reservations. A man can dodge a sauna for only so long before the word gets around.

We're covering the capital city of a country and it's quieter than central Mongolia. Andri Kjartansson, a personable paramedic who has been particularly welcoming, encourages me to stay in Reykjavik as long as I like.

'Since you arrived here it's never been so peaceful, you're a good omen,' he says.

I came to terms with this phenomenon early on. The most interesting work always seems to happen prior to my arrival or moments after I leave. Only yesterday, just before 8 am, Andri resuscitated a man found stuffed into a shopping trolley closely followed by a child drowned in the bath and then a car wrapped round a pole. Thirty minutes later I started my shift and we didn't turn the wheel for the rest of the day.

Still, I only half believe his stories. Downtown Reykjavik is a long way from the favelas of Rio. There is so little violence here the police don't carry guns and the city boasts the lowest crime rate in Europe. Even the occasional drunk we're dispatched to wake up on weekend nights would rather cuddle us than fight. With a population of a hundred and twenty who spend their winters indoors and their summers out of town, what could possibly go wrong?

At half-past five my beeper sounds and I carefully creep from my hiding place like a rabbit from its burrow once the hunter has gone. My uniform is a fluorescent yellow and blue jumpsuit over a rescue T-shirt formerly belonging to a medic who broke his neck in a cycling accident. How impractical it would be, I think, to get out of a sauna and into a jumpsuit on the clock.

When I reach the plant room I find Andri and his partner Björn Birgisson already have the engine running. In the time it's taken me to go down a fire pole these men have exited a sauna, pulled on their clothes, zipped up their boots and are waiting for me impatiently. Sixty seconds is all they get to be out the door, regardless of whether it's a heart attack or a leg cramp. Repeated failures to make this time result in a private interview with management. What an exhausting way of doing business.

'We're going to sweat all the way to the job,' predicts Andri as his partner flicks through ten different siren settings and opts for something classical.

Sweating *to* the job and *on* the job, I think to myself. Ólafur Ingólfsson, the last paramedic I worked with, perspired so heavily when he was dragged from the gymnasium that his forehead dripped like a leaking tap onto the patient.

'Hey, where were you anyway?' asks Andri.

When he gave me a tour of the station's state-of-the-art gymnasium on my first day, Andri convinced me the sauna, with its tiered Roman seating and room enough for a dozen men, was the centerpiece of the complex. The country is a refrigerator, he told me, and hot steam is vital.

But already I take a daily hot shower in geothermal water from the tap at the apartment I share with Kass and our newborn daughter, Paloma. One of the benefits of living in Iceland is this pleasure of bathing at home in mineral-rich natural spring water. Some say it is the reason Icelandic women are so beautiful, while others reckon one can always pick an Icelander by the pervading scent of sulphur that follows them about.

'Getting naked in public is not my thing,' I say.

'Getting naked? What's wrong with getting naked? We love getting naked! It's not like we're *fond* of each other, if that's what you're suggesting.'

My explanation to Andri is that most Australian blokes feel that saunas are generally run by, and for, homosexual men. And because Australian men tend to reaffirm their heterosexuality to one another through ultra-masculine modes of behaviour, any association with a sauna is strictly taboo.

Then there is the issue of taking my clothes off in front of fellow paramedics. As many of my colleagues back home are women, this could be a little awkward.

'Tell me, it isn't a matter of penis size, is it?' asks Andri hesitantly.

'Penis size?' I sound as surprised as I can. 'Oh no, no way, not at all, man.'

But he's probably right. After all, penis size is central to the perception of manhood anywhere, and I wouldn't be the only man to stress about a workplace sauna. Our job is intimate enough already, trapped in the front cabin of an ambulance with the same companion for months on end. The last thing we want to do in our downtime is strip off and sit in a little room together, all hot and sweaty and breathing heavily. As for taking a sauna with Icelandic medics, they would naturally consider me a representative of Australia. Both potential outcomes of a subtle scrutiny are most unsatisfactory. Should an unspoken penis comparison be in my favour, it would clearly put my hosts to shame, something I'm not in the habit of doing. And if, on the other hand, I came out second best, what a poor reflection on my nation.

'Just think of me!' says my wife Kass when I later share my dilemma with her. But I shake my head. Nothing good can possibly come from taking a sauna here and I'll do my utmost to avoid it.

We ascend a narrow stairwell smelling of laundry powder and cigarettes. The call is to someone having a fit and our response time has been so quick we find the epileptic still thrashing about on the kitchen floor, the back of her head banging up and down on the linoleum. Her jaw is locked in trismus and her face is red and puffed. It's a particularly violent tonic/clonic seizure and it's evident she needs 10 milligrams of Stesolid, the benzodiazepine sedative preferred by Icelandic paramedics. It's a difficult venture though, injecting a patient intravenously while arms and legs are doing the horizontal chicken dance. We give it a go all the same. Björn takes her right arm while I trap her left wrist between my knees, moving the sharp end of my cannula back and forth with the contracting of her elbow, trying to line up a vein. A couple of wayward punctures later and neither of us are in.

'Start with an IM,' says Andri calmly.

Björn draws up an intramuscular shot and stabs it into the woman's deltoid like a dart. I imagine this will satisfy Andri, who is running the call. But for him it's a half-measure. Known for his decisive and aggressive treatment, Andri turns the woman's head ever so slightly to the side and pins her jugular vein in one fell swoop.

I'm astonished. Never have I seen a jugular cannulation performed on a fitter.

Andri notices my reaction and chuckles. He attaches a loaded syringe and pushes in a bolus of anticonvulsant. Within seconds the woman stops fitting. Her face and mouth relax and her lungs replenish themselves with oxygen in deep, gasping breaths.

Later at the hospital other crews tease Andri about his cannula, implying he chose the external jugular for my benefit alone, something only a show-off would do.

But Andri is dismissive. 'Read the protocol and you'll see it recommends an immediate dose of IV Stesolid for continued fitting.' Turning to me he adds, 'Paramedics don't forget about the jugular, they're scared of it. You saw, didn't you? It was sticking out, begging for a sixteen-gauge.'

I'm impressed by his boldness but try not to gush. Most epileptics eventually stop fitting of their own accord if given a chance. And the best chance one can give them is a leisurely response time. 'On the next occasion,' I quip, 'he ought to remain in the sauna a little longer.'

Back at the station I take a cup of coffee with Sveinbjorn Berentsson – 'Svenni' for short, thank goodness – and we discuss a new extrication method for vehicle rollovers known as the Norway Technique in which a vehicle is manually righted with the patient still restrained before extrication begins. On his laptop Svenni shows me photographs demonstrating the process taken during an exercise in heavy snow last winter on the outskirts of Reykjavik.

'Even if the car is not upside down and has simply left the road, into a ditch for example, it is better to tow the car back onto the road before extricating,' he says. 'It will be stable on a firm surface. Under snow there are too many hazards, like fissures and holes. Many of our roads, remember, go straight through the middle of lava fields.'

Outside major towns the task of rescue is performed by volunteers from ICE-SAR, the Icelandic Search and Rescue Association that shot to fame on CNN as the first emergency team to land in Haiti following the recent earthquake. The primary funding for this lifesaving service comes from the sale of firecrackers to the public in the lead-up to New Year's Eve. Ironically, during these celebrations much of the life-saving required is related to firecracker mishaps. But as millions of krona are raised, it's no wonder people turn a blind eye, as it were.

In Icelandic the word for ambulance is *Sjukrabill* and these are supplied countrywide by the Red Cross – or Raudi Krossin as it's known here – in order to maintain a standard between the volunteer outfits operating in remote areas and the paid staff of towns and cities. In Reykjavik, the fire and rescue service operates these ambulances. What interests me most about Icelandic ambulance services – and the reason for my visit – is their recent conversion from the Franco-German model of pre-hospital care to the Anglo-American model. Before this change, ambulances in Iceland had doctors onboard. In 2008, an assessment by the

Ministry for Health decided that doctors would be better utilised in hospitals where there was a shortage. While a doctor may see ten patients on the busiest of days working for the ambulance, the same doctor could well see fifty or more patients in a hospital. Prior to my visit I was convinced that such a conversion is near impossible to achieve due to entrenched public expectations. Nevertheless, Iceland has done it and done it well.

It all started when Icelandic emergency medical technician Larus Petersen travelled to America in 1994 and, of his own accord, enrolled in a paramedic course being run in the city of Pittsburgh. After intensive study and an onroad practicum, Petersen graduated and returned to Reykjavik ready to initiate skills many of the doctors he was supporting were reluctant to use outside their hospital comfort zones.

According to Svenni, who followed in Petersen's footsteps to Pittsburgh, the new paramedics returning with field experience from a high call-volume American metropolis were intimidating for the Icelandic doctors, many of whom were fresh out of medical school 'after reading for seven years'.

'Many had trouble with taking initiative and managing under stress,' Svenni says. 'We work in a difficult environment, in dirty, cramped, chaotic places with bad lighting and no assistance. We carried the doctors a lot, we covered their arses many times.'

By the year 2000, the Icelandic Fire and Rescue Service were sponsoring selected firefighters to get their paramedic training in the United States. Most candidates topped their courses and developed an excellent reputation with the City of Pittsburgh Emergency Medical Service (EMS). It became evident to many in the health department that the returning paramedics were more suited to the pre-hospital environment than the doctors under whom they had operated.

'With all due respect to our doctors,' says Svenni. 'Most of them think differently to us. They work slower, there's more reflection, consideration. This is good in a hospital situation but not always in the field. Consistency was an issue too. Each doctor did things in another way. Since the change we have better consistency of treatment.'

Although the Fire and Rescue Service played no part in the Health Ministry's decision, a number of disgruntled doctors put the reform in jeopardy by going to the press and predicting hundreds of deaths would result. It was already a significant adjustment for the people of Iceland to make without such inflammatory remarks, and the doctors behind this were quickly reprimanded.

In spite of all this, the public seemed satisfied that paramedics would be capable substitutes for doctors. At the very least they were willing to permit the experiment. As in most other Anglo-American systems, a medical director would licence paramedics to administer emergency pharmacology while a doctor at the hospital would be available to approve use of restricted drugs via a phone call. This is known as 'medical control', and while it has not been adopted in Australia and the United Kingdom, it remains common practice across the United States.

Proof of how effective the crossover was came a year later as a result of an independent study conducted by Reykjavik University. To the relief of the Capital District Fire and Rescue Service it showed that patient care had actually *improved* as a result of the change. Access to advanced life support was much quicker due to a higher number of paramedics being available than ever there were doctors, while scene times had dropped dramatically. These factors, together with a follow-up of patients treated by ambulance crews, led the researchers to find there had been a 7 per cent improvement in patient outcomes since the change, even if the report concluded this was 'no significant difference'.

'I do sympathise with the doctors,' adds Svenni. 'We all know the real issue for them was never about the impact on patient care. It was about good old-fashioned sleep. They liked their sleep, simple as that.'

And as I've discovered, too, Icelandic paramedics get some very restful nightshifts.

The following day I am rostered with Hannes Sverrir, as placid a paramedic as you can get. His face of faded scars contrasts with his intensely blue eyes. Although he may not be as boisterous as his peers, he is magic with his patients and creates an atmosphere of familiarity and caring that gives the impression he is always on the verge of embracing them.

Our morning has ticked away without incident and the only command from God – a controller's voice piped through a stationwide intercom – has been to alert duty crews to the lunch option – Beef Stroganov or Caesar Salad. They call it the 'decision of the day' and I know exactly what they mean. It's agony, this choosing of what to eat, and it plagues every paramedic I know. For many years I've reflected on this seemingly inexplicable contradiction among professionals employed for their abilities to act decisively and under pressure. It's the same reason soldiers returning home from wars in which they make life-and-death decisions find themselves incapable of selecting a box of cereal at the supermarket. And so, at any one time, in cities around the world, ambulances are driving from suburb to suburb, slowing past neon-lit fast food joints and restaurants – Chinese, Indian, Thai, Italian – sometimes in circles or back and forth, while the paramedics inside deliberate ceaselessly about what they fancy. Although the Icelandic emergency services may not be able to eradicate this neurosis completely, they have at least reduced the personal and organisational cost of it by supplying meals on station and offering just two simple options.

In private, a few days earlier, Hannes told me he had come

to ambulance work from a business background, an office job that was sending him mad with boredom, sitting in front of a computer all day, every day. Strangely though, he was never one for blood and guts. Still isn't.

'What about your time in Pittsburgh?' I asked him.

'Yeah,' he replied, 'that was difficult.'

Not far off midday a child has come off his pushbike. According to our mobile data terminal, the boy is moaning in pain and cannot get up. Doesn't sound like there's much in it, but Hannes' partner, Hinrik, floors the accelerator along Miklabraut anyway, squeezing as much excitement as he can out of a dull day.

The boy, a tubby kid of about ten, has somehow managed to embed the bike's handlebar in his lower abdomen. As Hannes pulls back the boy's bloodstained T-shirt he unveils a fistful of glistening intestines, like cocktail sausages.

The paramedic recoils.

We apply oxygen and carry the boy to our stretcher. Once inside the ambulance, Hannes passes Hinrik a packet of gauze and plastic flask of saline.

'Please, Hinrik,' he says, his face pale and contorted in disgust. 'Would you mind? Before we go?'

Hinrik smiles a knowing smile and Hannes steps out of the ambulance to take some audible inward breaths and calm his nerves at the roadside. How, indeed, he managed to pass his practicum in the United States with all those ghetto shootings is beyond me. His partner there must have worked double time.

In the Fire and Rescue Service dining room with panoramic views over Reykjavik, the only place left will have me sitting beside Deputy Chief Birgir Finnsson who is finishing off a plate of gelatinous chocolate soup and submerged crispbread. This, as it turns out, is not a dessert.

When I approach him with my Caesar salad he smiles and I know he knows I know what he will ask me. If Birgir hadn't made it his mission to get me into a sauna I'd probably spend more time with him. He's a very likeable family man. Kass and I, along with baby Paloma, have greatly enjoyed dinner in the company of his own charming wife and three young girls. We consider each other friends and I'm truly ashamed to be hiding from a friend. What a terrible and juvenile thing to do.

'It's an innocent social event,' he says directly. 'It's a place for swapping stories about accidents and emergencies, about running ambulances, you know, it's the reason you're here, isn't it? You'll enjoy it. I'll find you at 5 pm.'

Unlikely, I think to myself, as he gets up.

'Can't we discuss those subjects over lunch here?' I say, somewhat helplessly.

He laughs and shakes his head.

'Impossible!' Then leaning down to me, his voice now hushed, he adds, '*Everything* comes out in the sauna. *Truth* comes out in the sauna. Until you take one you'll never understand. Whenever it may be, you *will* take a sauna with us before leaving Iceland, *that* we'll make sure of.'

As I'm left there picking at my salad I think about all the man has done to welcome me, let alone the respect his position as Deputy Chief demands. How long can I avoid his invitation before I'm considered impolite? Indeed, if Birgir should corner me late in the afternoon, refusing him will be impossible.

By 4 pm I am out the door and on my way home.

Heavy rain in thick streams is pummelling the double-glass windows of the station when I arrive for work on Monday morning. Rain always comes sideways in Iceland, propelled by vicious polar winds blowing from the north. And they call this summer.

Hot coffee steams from the mugs of day shift crews as they do their monthly audit in the plant room, squinting at the fine print on the side of each glass ampoule for use-by dates, stocking up the crash drawers. Most have already had their porridge upstairs. One of the medics folds a little *neftobak* Icelandic nose tobacco into a small square of toilet tissue and pushes it under his top lip where the bulge will gradually release its stimulant effects while giving everyone the impression he has been recently whacked in the mouth. Most other medics prefer to snort the stuff, which they carry around in a grey, kidney-shaped bottle. Whatever the route of administration, it's an evil substance with the odour of a month-old corpse.

Two basic life support (BLS) medics, Palmi and Eirikur, who are rarely permitted to work together on account of their larrikinism, entertain us with a deadpan exchange about plastic surgery. Eirikur's sister has apparently procured herself a breast enlargement and the discussion centres around whether or not she would permit her own brother to 'have a squeeze'.

The crews laugh raucously while Andri shakes his head and Eirikur throws Palmi a dummy punch in defence of his sister's honour.

After making the 'decision of the day' – fish or pita – and marking it down in the book, I peruse the gallery of former fire chiefs painted in oils on metre-high canvases, each of them in the same pose, their faces dark and earnest. And then, as so often happens to me, one experience foreshadows the next.

An alert comes over the speakers, a chest pain for 701, the ambulance to which I'm assigned. We head out as Palmi curses the patients for calling whenever they hear his belly rumble.

'What are you talking about? You're always hungry!' retorts Andri.

Palmi grunts and throws the ambulance round a bend with a screeching of tyres.

Luckily, facing the street on the ground floor of a complex of luxury apartments from where the patient has called, the rear doors of a bakery are open and a rotund, troll-like pastry chef pokes his head out, wondering why an ambulance has reversed into his delivery dock. Stepping onto the street we are enveloped by the mouth-watering scent of fresh, piping-hot buns and can see them lined up on racks recently removed from the oven. The baker notices us eyeing off his bread while grabbing our gear and uses it to his advantage.

'Something going on?' he enquires.

Ambulance crews get this all the time, complete strangers assuming it's part of our job description to satisfy their curiosity. Normally we ignore them or smile and politely explain the case is confidential.

But the baker knows we are keen on his buns and I can tell he won't be giving any up unless he gets something back, some gossip fodder he can impress his customers with, or at least liven up his day a little.

'Maybe a heart attack,' says Palmi reluctantly.

'Oh,' says the baker. 'That's no good.'

As Palmi locks the ambulance the baker says, 'Here, have a bun.' He passes each of us a steaming bread roll, crisp on the outside and soft on the inside, just as a bun ought to be.

Chest pains are to a paramedic what buns are to a baker and this wouldn't be a case worth writing about were it not for the fact that I recognise the patient, or think I do. Meeting us at the door is an elderly gentleman in a dapper silver shirt with cufflinks, looking as if he has spent an hour grooming himself before calling us. Andri introduces himself and beckons the man to sit in the nearest chair and not to move. Even a few steps in cases of complete heart failure can spell the end for some. By turning on the hall light I get a better look at the man and, while Palmi is prepping an ECG, I ask the man, 'Sir, you're the former Fire Chief of Reykjavik, aren't you?'

He looks taken aback, not only because I've addressed him in English, but surprised I've recognised him at all. Andri and Palmi are equally astonished.

'Your portrait,' I say. 'I saw it this morning.'

He seems flattered and as pleased as anyone would be to hear it mentioned.

'Yes, took the artist days to paint it.'

'It didn't have a name under it though,' I tell him.

'I know, a pity that. My name is Rúnar Bjarnason.'

Bjarnason has been suffering chest pains since the beginning of July and only now decided to call.

'Typical fireman,' Andri whispers to me before squirting some nitro-lingual spray into the man's mouth. Neither Andri nor Palmi recognised the old chief.

Bjarnason seems eager to tell me about the early days.

'When I started as fire chief in 1966, an ambulance may as well have been transporting potatoes. We only got our first acute care ambulance in 1983. Can you believe it? But look at the service now,' he says, beaming. 'Just look at it!'

Palmi prints off a twelve-lead strip, which shows a possible anteroseptal infarct. But, oh, how impressed is Bjarnason to see the monitor flashing and buzzing and issuing commands in its cold monotone.

Frequently, when the rescuer is in need of being rescued, he is tragically let down and disappointed. A car accident I had on the way to work in Newcastle some years ago convinced me of this. As I lay slumped over the steering wheel gasping for breath with blood soaking my uniform and watching smoke issue forth from a bonnet crumpled to the windscreen, I saw the first ambulance approach the scene, crawl past for a brief look then disappear again down the road. Apparently they were tasked to see a 'more serious' case elsewhere. Likewise, other colleagues have had family members collapse and waited far too long for help. You give your all, for years on end, and when your own turn comes – disappointment. But Rúnar Bjarnson is beaming with pride. How satisfying it must be for him, I say, to receive this advanced treatment from a service he himself helped set in motion. While most of us build families that will make our end years joyous and others accumulate wealth for a lavish retirement, Bjarnson's investment is giving him a longer life.

Going out the door, Andri's face drops.

'Oh shit,' he whispers.

'What is it?' I ask.

My colleague stands behind the stretcher as we wait for the lift, his back against the wall. 'Look what I'm wearing! Socks in sandals, for crying out loud! I forgot to put my boots on. That's *never* happened before. Unbelievable!'

At the station, ambulance and fire crews get around in sandals, slippers and clogs, only pulling on their rescue boots when heading to a case. Andri looks devastated.

'Just my luck, the one and only time I go out with socks in sandals and we get the former fire chief. Do you think he noticed?'

I can imagine in Rúnar Bjarnson's day they not only *wore* their boots but polished them every morning. For the rest of the job Andri slinks around trying to hide his casual footwear.

Later, other paramedics tell me that despite his achievements the old chief was strict and inflexible and led a service into the nineties with management techniques decades out of date. Most remarkable to me is that the man could have been fire chief for more than twenty years.

Jón Viðar Matthíasson, the current fire chief, on the other hand, is adored by all. His primary concern, they tell me, is the welfare of his staff and each one of them has his private mobile number in their phones. I suspect the CEOs of larger emergency services might find this idea a little daunting. The sheer sumptuousness of station facilities, the gymnasiums and bedrooms and lounges and satellite televisions are an example of Matthíasson's passionate belief that staff morale and emotional wellbeing is the key to efficient service delivery. Rarely have I come across emergency service CEOs who make it their habit, as he does, to meet his crews once a week and buy them hotdogs. The hotdog, as it happens, is Iceland's most popular snack, introduced to the country by US troops stationed here during World War II. At that time, American forces outnumbered the population of Reykjavik and brought such prosperity to the country that locals still refer to World War II as 'the lovely war'. Most appreciated of all were the hotdogs, and soon after taking the old fire chief to hospital we are sitting with the current fire chief eating them during a casual debriefing. It's a perfect opportunity to thank him for loaning my family a Subaru station wagon belonging to the service and I tell him we plan to explore the area around the Eyjafjallajökull volcano and the adjacent glacier the next week.

This prompts a discussion of the eruption that stopped European air traffic in 2010, the most exciting moment in recent history for emergency workers in Iceland. While the rest of the world imagined all hell had broken loose on the island and prayed for the people and their poor emergency services, it did not reflect the reality of the local conditions. Because Eyjafjallajökull is situated on the far south coast of the country and the wind bears south-east for much of the year, the cloud of ash and fine glass particles blew away from Iceland and only a single farmstead at the base of the volcano was affected. Ironically, Icelandair continued to fly when all other airlines in Europe were grounded.

Once it was established that the glacial melt caused by the volcanic heat would not result in major flooding, many firemen and paramedics simply took time off and drove out to camp beside the magma. Even Deputy Chief Finnsson tells me he spent a night reclining in his 4x4 beside a burning river of molten rock and a hundred-foot fountain of bubbling gold so beautiful he couldn't take his eyes off it to sleep.

Meanwhile, back in Reykjavik, the disaster control room had instead become a busy media unit with hundreds of phone lines ringing off the hook. There were calls from prime ministers and airlines and businesses around Europe, many abusing the Icelandic emergency services for not doing more, as if it was within their power to extinguish an active volcano. Absurdly, as the ash cloud spread and the number of calls increased, ordinary firemen were taken off the road to answer telephones.

Extra staff are required for Iceland's wildest annual music festival taking place on Heimaey, the largest of the Westman Islands – or Vestmannaeyjar – off the southern coast of the country, not far from Eyjafjallajökull. Here, more than ten thousand punters pitch their tents on the floor of a dormant volcano where a giant stage is erected for bands playing from dusk until dawn. Nowhere in the world, I'm told, are people as reckless with booze as they are on this particular weekend in Vestmannaeyjar. It's where Icelanders lose their virginity and return to their Viking selves. There is even a 'rape squad' of burly female volunteers who patrol the site armed with torches and batons.

To reach it I take a half-hour Air Iceland flight packed with youth clutching clinking plastic bags of vodka bottles, casks of wine and slabs of Polar Beer. By the time we've reached cruising altitude, the flight has turned into a mile-high dance party. Regrettably, I've come dressed as a paramedic and spend my time declining quality liquor. A uniform doesn't deter the pilot, however, who proves he is clearly in the spirit of things by doing a daring swoop along the cliffs of Heinaey to a chorus of excitable screams from his now fully inebriated passengers.

At the tiny airport I'm met by an off-duty fireman in a neck-brace who laughs and points at the yellow digits printed on the sleeve of my rescue T-shirt.

'Number 22! That's me, I'm number 22! That's my shirt you're wearing!'

Inconceivable. It's the guy who broke his neck. He's off work, but A-okay for boozing at a festival. As for strange coincidences, these are occurring so frequently I fear I might become immune to them and lose my astonishment.

'Sorry Number 22, they only *lent* it to me.'

'No, no, it's fine. You can have it. I'll get a new one.'

He appears more pleased about contributing a souvenir to an international guest than I am about wearing a second-hand T-shirt belonging to a wheelchair-bound fireman.

At a suburban house where medical crews are being billeted I join paramedic Njalli Palsson – his first name pronounced 'Nelly' – his paramedic partner Hlynr Hoskuldsson – who suggests I just call him 'Lenny' – and a couple of intermediate life support (ILS) medics, Óskar and Dagur. Before we begin the shift there is soft drink and pizza all round and when Njalli passes me a slice I notice he is wearing a gold ring depicting the moulded insignia of a square and compass. So much for the secrecy of the freemasons, I point out. What about all those passwords and grips?

'We're a society with secrets, not a secret society,' he says, a little irritated. 'Obviously you're not a freemason.'

'No.'

'It's worth looking into, it will make you a better man.'

My Australian grandfather, I've been told, was once a member of a Lodge in Sydney, though I've never been into clubs myself, especially those where grown men don aprons and conduct rituals with swords. Humans taking themselves too seriously have always had a paradoxical effect on me and I doubt I'd last ten minutes without bursting into a fit of giggles.

'Are there many of you in the service?' I ask Njalli.

'Many masons? Working in ambulances?'

I nod.

'Yes, there are.'

'How many?'

He pauses for a moment.

'Let's just say there are many. Pizza?'

It may not be the case anymore, but there was a time when ambulance services in every state of Australia were also heavy with freemasons and it was generally believed that a promotion was only possible via that secret handshake.

'What about females in the job?' I ask Njalli.

The paramedic guesses where I'm going and smiles.

'No objection,' he says.

I'm not convinced, and when I learn from Birgir Finnsson that the service currently has no serving females my suspicions were confirmed. The Capital District Fire and Rescue Service is quite plainly a boy's club. Unlike the Islamic Republic of Pakistan, Iceland can't use cultural or religious sensitivity as an excuse. What it could use, I suppose, is the 5 pm sauna. How would the service possibly include females without frightening them off on the first day?

'It's a tricky subject,' said Finnsson when I push the matter in his office. 'You see, on our last intake we had one hundred applications and only three were from women. Even after lowering the fitness benchmark, none of them could pass the basic requirements. What do I do? Naturally I would like to have females in this job. But how far do we compromise on the fitness criteria to achieve it?'

A lack of female paramedics and a macho atmosphere on station are perhaps the unavoidable side-effects of ambulance services run by fire departments. As every medic must also be a firefighter and adhere to the physical standards of one, it automatically excludes individuals whose strengths are more intellectual than physical. To counter this problem some fire departments in the United States make it possible for recruits to select an EMS career without having to be a firefighter. This would appear to be the sensible strategy as the firefighter/medic has always seemed a contradiction to me. While firefighters run towards a fire, clever medics sensibly run the other way.

Back by the volcano, I spend most of the night huddled in the front seat of the ambulance while a biting wind laced with ice batters the tents of the merrymakers, none of whom seem the slightest bit cold. Blonde girls in plaits swig Viking ale on basalt boulders while teenagers in orange rubber fisherman trousers worn high over thick knitted jumpers wrestle in the damp grass. Not one of these Icelanders shiver or rub their arms or crouch with their back to the wind. Not one of them flinches from the cold, even for a second. Hours of sing-a-longs keep the crowds happy, though everyone is slightly disappointed puffin hunting has been banned this year. Apparently the island is famous for its freshly extracted puffin hearts, swallowed whole. Still, there is ample booze to compensate.

At the opposite end of the crater from where the all-night concert is taking place, a tin hut the size of a public toilet is serving as a makeshift clinic. Here we park the ambulances and take turns working through a queue of happy loud-mouthed teenagers presenting their minor wounds like festival souvenirs. We take turns because seasoned paramedics have little more than fifteen minutes of tolerance for grossly intoxicated people, even if they want to kiss and hug us and shake our hands with sticky palms and tell us three inches from our faces that we're their best friends in the whole wide world.

Paralytic drunks are a different matter. The plan for these patients appears ingenious and inhumane in equal measure and involves a giant shipping container into which they are heaped side by side like tuna. Western city hospitals over-exposed to alcohol abuse would surely find such a strategy appealing given that emergency departments are perpetually congested with people sleeping off the grog. Meanwhile my friends insist the 'drunk dump' is the police department's idea and not officially endorsed by medics. Whatever the case, it occurs to me there are few better ways for the inebriated to stay warm than to share body heat with one another in the confines of the most wind-resistant structure available. Indeed, during the night a guy comes to my cabin window and tells me he's been lying in his tent 'like a starfish' for three hours trying to stop it from leaving the ground.

At this time of year the country gets about half an hour of semi-darkness around midnight, dark enough in the opinion of festival organisers for a quick fireworks display. As rockets explode from a pulpit of rock I notice they don't have much height about them. Heavy booming like thunder ricochets round the walls of the crater – it's so loud and enveloping one could easily imagine that the volcano has awoken after a million years. Flashes of colour glance off the highest ridges and showers of light rain down, glowing and flickering to the ground. Before long, the crater is so thick with smoke the fireworks are no longer visible and I begin to cough violently.

I hear a cry go up and one of the paramedics suddenly pulls the side door of the ambulance open, unclips the latch of a fire extinguisher and runs off with it. I stumble out and follow him. Just over a rise of gnarled lava a large tent is well alight. People frantically unpeg surrounding tents while a half-naked couple are comforting each other in shock, suggesting their tent may have been hot enough already. Amazingly, once the fire is out everyone opens another beer and calmly disperses.

By 5 am the shift has proven no worse than any Saturday night in Sydney, London or New York. Only here the kids are sleeping it off in a billowing tent city battered by an arctic gale that threatens to snap-freeze my entire body whenever I step out of the ambulance.

Before taking some rest ourselves we sit with the sun on our faces in a yard of snow-white clover protected from the wind by neighbouring houses. Hlynr, who has worn his Pittsburgh EMS baseball cap all night, passes around pieces of brittle dried haddock for breakfast. Njalli offers Óskar and me a Café Crème cigarillo. Sleep deprivation and time to relax with my colleagues prompts me to ask about the station sauna.

'Oh, how I love that sauna,' says Hlynr.

The others nod and mumble in agreement, their eyes squinted shut in the sunlight.

It's the right time to be frank, I think to myself.

'Sauna's not my thing really,' I say.

'The heat bothers you?' asks Njalli.

'No, no … it's more about the nudity, I suppose. We don't do much nudity back home, not like that.'

They're surprised to hear it.

'What about change rooms at swimming pools?'

'I go to the beach mostly.'

'So?'

'So, I'm not familiar with the etiquette. I mean, is it like visiting a public toilet, you avoid looking left or right, maintain tunnel vision and all that?'

Njalli and the others chuckle and Hlynr says, 'We Icelanders, we know we're hung like monsters, there's no need to check and make sure.'

How reassuring.

Already I'm unsettled by the prevalence among Icelandic rescue workers of nicknames like Tripod, Anaconda and Javelin. There's even a Totem and a bloody Torpedo.

'If you need to prepare yourself,' adds Hlynr, 'you may have to Google.'

'Google what?'

'Icelandic penis, Viking cock, I don't know. Prepare yourself, and you decide.'

My cigarillo seems all the shorter after our conversation, though I've hardly puffed on it.

Hlynr may have a point, yet the only access to the internet I get is at the Reykjavik Headquarters and I dread the idea of being caught searching for Icelandic penis. No doubt this would make my attendance at any future 5 pm sauna even more complicated than it's already become.

Because the names of Icelandic people are almost as unpronounceable as the country's volcanoes, I'm relieved most have simplified versions for the foreign guest or when they are travelling. Oddly, a lanky paramedic with a deadpan sense of humour by the name of Stefán has shortened his name to 'Stebbi' despite Stefán being the most sensible first name I've encountered here.

So I'm back in Reykjavik on shift with Stebbi and his partner, a young ILS medic by the name of Gudjon Gudmundsson who, in contrast to Stebbi, has a face fixed with a constant grin. He also uses the Icelandic word for 'yes' – spelt 'ja' but pronounced 'yow' – peppered among his English. It's the Friday night after Vestmannaeyjar and as we cruise the main drag downtown nothing seems to be going on. Stebbi is recounting the spike in suicides after the *kreppa* when many in Iceland lost everything.

'It was like the most creative suicide competition,' says Stebbi. 'One guy killed himself by taking a whale meat barbecue inside his apartment, closing the doors and windows and waiting till the barbecue chewed up all the oxygen.'

After turning past a billboard advertising the Icelandic ice-cream company Emmessis – which in English medical terms means 'vomit' – Gudjon raises the subject of saunas without any provocation, mentioning the sauna obsession of the Finns and how the sauna is a Finnish invention and how glad I ought to be that I'm not working on the ambulances of Finland.

'Once,' says Gudjon, 'when I belonged to the Icelandic Boy Scouts, I went to an international scout jamboree in Thailand and the Finnish Boy Scouts were there too and you know what they brought along with them?'

'Let me guess, a sauna?'

'Yow, but not just any sauna. They had a damn *tent* sauna.'

'Tent sauna?'

'Sauna in a tent.'

'How can you have a sauna in a tent?'

He looks at Stebbi then back at me.

'Zip it up good,' he says.

What intrigues me more than the existence of a tent sauna is why the Finns would consider it necessary in Thailand. The place is a sauna anyway.

Adjacent to the plaza there is a bright American-style fast-food joint and we pull in for burgers and fries. Waiting at the counter, Stebbi and Gudjon speak of their appreciation of Australian films. At the time of its release in 1993, one of our darkest cinematic exports – Rolf De Heer's *Bad Boy Bubby* – was so popular among ambulance workers in Iceland they started a fan club.

Now it's football, Aussie Rules no less.

A week earlier I went to see The Ravens, the Icelandic Aussie Rules team, train on a windswept soccer field surrounded by grey volcanic formations and dreary apartment blocks. White-blond men with smooth Nordic faces sprinted back and forth wearing the tops and short shorts for which the sport is famous. Despite the skewed kicking and frequent ball-dropping I could only marvel at how this football game could end up being embraced by a nation on the opposite side of the planet, and just how well the Icelandic Aussie Rules team had done to be competing internationally after only a couple of years.

Just as we're about to take a bite from our burgers, the beeper goes. I look across the table at my hosts. Their burgers are halfway to their mouths, as is mine, and for a millisecond I wonder what they will do. But like the rest of the crews, they are firefighters first, paramedics second. Both put their burgers down and get up.

Normally, back in Sydney, I'd at least steal a bite at this point, or, depending on the case in question, eat the whole bloody thing – few individuals are better able to consume takeaway meals in a matter of seconds than hungry paramedics. But the boys have not done this. No, it's 2100 hours and we're all starving and we all know the outcome of the call will most likely be unaffected by the twenty seconds it takes to down a hamburger, but they leave their food behind all the same. They leave it getting cold in polystyrene boxes full of fries already flaccid. Do I follow their lead, abandoning my own entrenched work habits, or do I revert to what I know is most sensible, for my own wellbeing and that of the patient who will benefit from a happy and well-nourished paramedic?

I take a bite and head for the door.

An ILS crew has called for assistance and we park beside their ambulance in the sleepy cul-de-sac of Haaleitisbraut. For at least a couple of days, while his neighbours have been going about their business, an old man has been dragging himself through his apartment, naked, in agony and slowly dying. Unable to reach him by phone, the man's son called an ambulance.

It's a stomach-turning scene. The carpet from one end of the house to the other is smeared with a putrid trail of black excrement, the hallmark of a gastrointestinal haemorrhage. This unpleasant mix of blood and bile and shit is known as *malena* and is often described as the colour of coffee grounds, which, as a connoisseur of good coffee, I consider a dismaying comparison. The *malena* is long dry, but in the corner where the first crew is loading the man onto a stretcher the stuff looks relatively fresh. The patient's entire body, I observe, is also slathered in it.

'He's pretty sick,' says Óskar, the medic on the other ambulance with whom I spent time in Vestmannaeyar. I recognise his partner Birkir as the man who picked us up from Keflavik airport.

'Where were you guys?' he says.

Stebbi makes the brief charade of a hamburger stopping on the way to his mouth and Óskar smiles. Then Stebbi asks for a GCS, referring to the patient's level of consciousness, using the universal Glasgow Coma Scale.

As far as Óskar can ascertain it's a plain three-out-of-fifteen. This is, oddly enough, the lowest possible score a person can get and one that indicates profound unconsciousness. As for his blood pressure, it's impalpable.

Four of us are crammed into the back of the ambulance, stepping over kit bags and each other's feet. Óskar looks for a vein in the man's left *cubital fossa* and I snap an oxygen mask onto his face, noticing that our patient is making very little respiratory effort. It then appears, on closer inspection, he has stopped breathing altogether.

'Respiratory arrest,' I tell Stebbi, who is already setting up for an intubation.

Everyone looks at the monitor in time to see a bradycardia turning into a slow, unrecognisable rhythm that will likely dwindle away in the next minute.

'Pulse?' enquires Stebbi.

My fingers go to the man's carotid.

'Nothing,' I say. It appears the man is clinically dead.

'CPR,' says Stebbi calmly, not that I don't already know the drill, but someone has to 'run the arrest', as we say. While an orchestra can play without a conductor, it never sounds quite as tight.

Birkir clenches his hands together and places them over the man's sternum, pumping up and down at a rate of 100 beats per minute, or, as the medics here find helpful, the tempo of the disco anthem 'Stayin' Alive'. More appropriate, in my opinion, would be 'The Final Countdown' by Europe. But in 2008 the American Heart Association in conjunction with the University of Illinois officially recommended the Bee Gees hit as the best way for students of resuscitation to perfect the speed of compressions. Given that every paramedic here seems to have the latest issue of the American *Journal of Emergency Medical Services* (JEMS) lying around his home, clinical advances and technical fads are frequently incorporated into Icelandic emergency care.

While hyperventilating the patient in the seconds before Stebbi sinks the tube I glance at Birkir stooping over doing CPR and he asks for my feedback. The patient is no longer cyanosed, I tell him, a pretty good sign. But moments later Birkir gets better proof than a patient's colour can offer him, a proof so terrible it has petrified some of the toughest paramedics in the game.

In a slow and chilling motion, the patient's left hand rises off the floor of the ambulance where it has limply hung, rises like the hand of a puppet, sliding up the inner thigh of Birkir's right leg.

'My God ...' says Birkir, turning pale but continuing bravely with his CPR. 'My God! Is this normal? Is this normal? Guys!'

There is panic in his eyes but before he can say or do anything more the patient has taken a firm grip of his rescuer's crotch. Seeing the horror unfold, Stebbi brings an immediate halt to the proceedings.

'Okay, stop compressions,' he orders.

The man's arm drops down again.

'Check for a pulse.'

It's not the first time I've encountered such a thing. On rare occasions in witnessed cardiac arrests and with highly effective chest compressions, a patient's brain may be oxygenated enough to produce a motor or even verbal response. Birkir has been in the job less than two years and this is all too much for him. Braced against a wall of the ambulance he mops his brow with a towel, shaken by the ball-grabber.

'Damn good compressions,' Stebbi says with a chuckle.

The man has a pulse, an outcome that rarely occurs with CPR alone. But this is no coronary. It's an absolute hypovolaemia, a state of low blood volume due to internal bleeding. With posture, fluid replacement and CPR the guy has been scraped back from the brink of death and all of us feel rather pleased with ourselves.

As proven by the likes of superstar Björk and band Sigur Ros, extraordinary musical talent is in high concentration in Iceland and, until volcanic eruptions and bank collapses, the country was perhaps most famous for its music, much of which Kass and I call 'snow folk'. Icelanders, from tradesmen to paramedics, seem to be teaching themselves a new instrument, performing at concerts or recording albums. And so it is entirely natural that an ode to the shit-covered, ball-grabbing gentleman we revived is plucked out later that night by Birkir on his acoustic guitar using the same hands that had brought the man back to life. Accompanying him is shift manager Hafsteinn Halldorsson who produces, to our surprise, a purple ukulele. What it is with volcanic islands and ukuleles I do not know. But a gentle, dreamlike atmosphere ensues as they serenade Stebbi and Gudjon and the rest of the nightshift with ancient Icelandic folk duets until everyone begins nodding off right there where they sit despite the nose tobacco that should be keeping them up.

In the morning, over porridge, I remind my colleagues that few of their counterparts in other capital cities of the world would have slept right through a Friday night as we have just done. Don't write that in your book, whatever you do, they joke. Besides, it's not always like this and I'm the one responsible. If only the boss would pay me a wage to spend every nightshift at their station in order to guarantee peace and quiet. Unfortunately for these men I am nearing the end of my stay and Monday is set to be my last shift in Iceland.

The day proves as uneventful as most other Mondays in Reykjavik. Over the intercom at 8 am the choices are announced – fillet-of-fish or braised pork – once again the most challenging decision these paramedics are likely to make all day. The amount of downtime is not important. After all, it's Iceland, not Iraq, and it's a mistake to be critical of an emergency service for not being busy enough. Services that keep their paramedics working by sending them on routine transfers leave areas uncovered and put lives at risk. Better it is that medics twiddle their thumbs for a whole day if it means a rapid response to that cardiac arrest at the end of it. With good reason, the public will judge an ambulance service on its ability to respond quickly rather than the number of patients it can take from one clinic to another.

At the stroke of 5 pm as I help myself to fruit salad brought to the station by the wife of the shift manager, a tradition among the fire and ambulance personnel of Iceland, Deputy Finnsson turns up in his gym shorts.

'Okay, Aussie, let's go,' he says.

The day crews lying back on lounges know this is crunch time and so do I. All of them wish me luck. As I'm led down the spiral iron staircase, down the corridor to the sauna, it's as if I've been on death row, my execution constantly postponed until now. Isn't this what they call 'the final walk'? Through one security door after another I approach the chamber of my demise until I stand in the change room beside the communal showers adjacent to Iceland's Fire and Rescue Service sauna. Before I know it the deputy has his kit off and is looking my way expectantly, wondering perhaps if I will make a desperate last-minute run for it.

But there is no turning back. Not now.

Without further pause, I unzip my jumpsuit.

DEATH IN VENICE

Italy

As we round the end of the Fondamenta Nuove, before we disappear into the narrow canals of Cannaregio, Dr Manuela Silvestri points to the horizon where the Dolomites are still white-tipped on the first day of an Italian summer. Behind us, coming over the Lido, a storm is bearing down, growling like Saint Mark's winged lion. With its hind legs in water and front legs on land, it is the emblem of the Venetian ambulance boats belonging to SUEM – an *acronimo* for Servizio di Urgenza Emergenza Medica. Around us the electricity of pent-up lightning prickles the skin while our siren echoes along the ancient walls rising out of tourmaline waters. Our wake follows us in a foaming wave coursing above the waterline marked by dark-green algae on the weathered stone. Moored boats are tossed about like driftwood. A furious wind rushes over my cheeks and I'm sprayed with water, ducking like the others under the last bridge. When Emiliano, our young *pilota*, shoots out onto the Grand Canal in a fountain of whitewash, my stomach drops and my body drums with adrenalin. Not since I first started as a medic has responding to a case thrilled me this much. While millions of tourists pay a hundred euro an hour to inch through the minor canals, I'm seeing the most stunning city on earth at forty knots, free of charge.

Pity about the hair, though.

Styling my 1950s pompadour is no easy feat. It's as close to Elvis as permissible for a medic, thanks to Tony, my talented Sydney barber. While nowadays it only takes me five minutes in the morning, a decent gust of wind can ruin it completely. And rain signals further disaster. I only mention this because the glamorous *Dottoressa* Manuela has the same trouble. When not at work, she keeps the appearance and grace of a Cinecitta movie star, a classy belladonna in the model of Sophia Loren, with broad designer sunglasses, high-waisted dresses and long, elegant cigarettes. Working on ambulance boats is a particular challenge for a lady like her. Earlier in the week she swore at the advent of a light rain shower and we found our common ground.

'*Merda!* Can you believe it, Benjamino? I'm spending *cinquantaquattro* euros a week on my hair thanks to this job!'

Tony charges me less because I'm his friend. But I certainly know where Manuela's coming from. Venetian canals are, quite simply, hostile to the hair. Mid-July is a hot blow dryer. Or it rains. Winters are even worse for rain, not to mention the snow. I told her if I'm ever caught in rain back home I try and send a junior officer out to check the patient. Hearing this she laughed, clapping her hands with delight.

'*Bravo! Si, anche a me!* Also, also! If there is case in open place, boys will bring to me inside boat, everything we can do here, no?'

An ambulance worker's bad hair can be as devastating to patients as incorrect treatment. One of the primary objectives of the rescuer is to achieve immediate and total credibility in order to gain the patient's confidence. Seconds may count in emergency care, but so do first impressions. Sadly, personal appearance has never been a key performance indicator. From the white tracksuits and Dunlop Volleys of German medics to the loose and faded jumpsuits issued to Australians, it's obvious that a focus on clinical development has forced personal presentation into the back seat. To a patient, their rescuer's in-depth knowledge of anatomy and physiology is, for the most part, hidden. What is not hidden is the rescuer's uniform and grooming. Knowing Latin prefixes may be well and good, but they matter far less to a patient in distress than the comfort of believing they are in competent hands. And this competency is conveyed as much by appearance as it is by manner and care.

Approaching the Rialto Bridge we are the greatest attraction in Venice. Hundreds of faces peer over the famous stone *ponte*. They stop and turn on both sides of the Grand Canal and wave from the plush bellies of gondolas. Emiliano, a former pilot with the Venetian fire brigade, carves up the surface of the canal. Looking back, I see a dozen gondoliers struggling to keep their bounty of tourists afloat over the waves we've left behind.

No one goes this fast in Venice. In the smaller canals where the speed limit is set at five kilometres per hour, even ambulances cannot travel quicker. Here a wake too high can rush through the alleys and knock people off their feet. Small boats may be capsized, houses flooded. More serious still is the risk of collision. And stopping for traffic at these intersections of water is much harder to do in a boat than in a car on land. Even Emiliano has had near misses. Operating boats in Venice is considered a fine art and a pilot's reputation is highly valued. Big accidents are thus quite rare. But even minor collisions can be costly, particularly when it comes to gondolas. Just last week, an ambulance barely nudged a gondola and the damage came to 4000 euros.

When he heard about that accident, Emiliano said, 'Maybe I drive fast, but never near a gondola. We are at their mercy here in Venice.'

At their mercy?

Is it not true that no vehicle on land or water has right of way over an ambulance, unless of course it belongs to a presidential convoy? In which case even ambulances heading to a heart attack cannot cross its path without risking a bullet.

'In your country everyone pulls over for an ambulance, right? In Venice, my friend, *we* pull over for the gondola.'

Of the four hundred or so gondoliers in Venice, most are from the same extended family. Pretty as they are lounging about on every little bridge in their blue-and-white shirts and hats gaily adorned with ribbons, I don't like them at all. I don't like the straw boater that takes me back to my days at a Sydney private school where the uniform hasn't changed in a hundred years. I don't like the way they look at Kass when she passes them. I don't like their oily, distasteful charm. And I don't like how they drool for the next throng of American girls ready for seduction or the next wad of cash from a Japanese wallet. I've been told that to be born a gondolier is to be born into money, that they earn more than almost everybody else in the city. Money buys power and in this upside-down world power has right of way. Looking down from the Rialto Bridge one may frequently observe fully laden *vaporettos* coming to a complete standstill for a single passing gondola.

Were they like the mafia, I wanted to know?

Emiliano smiled and replied, 'You could say that, if you chose to say that,' which in Venetian terms is ample confirmation.

In Venice, every ambulance pilot is a rugged seafarer. Some of them began as gondoliers themselves, rowing sick people to hospital in the late 1950s, the ringing of a brass bell heralding their approach. This was half a century after the invention of the motorboat. Venice, however, is not a place where things evolve quickly. Back then the service was known as the Croce Azzurra – the Blue Cross – before it came under the command of the hospital system. Most of the pilots are still tanned, fit, muscular men with Sailor Jerry-style tattoos of anchors and mermaids on broad arms. One fellow even has a tattoo of an eight-pointed compass rose, like those found on nautical charts.

Keys to their boats are attached to little circular corks in case they are dropped in the water, though I've never seen a careless pilot. On the contrary, they are masters of the Venetian waterways. Like ancient mariners who intimately knew the winds and stars of an open sea, Venetian ambulance pilots are alert to the tides and depths of each canal, the height of bridges and the width of water corridors too narrow for boats or leading to nowhere. Even on the waist-deep lagoon where few of the underwater trenches are marked by wooden piles known as *briccole*, the boatmen are able to execute the speediest of turns at precisely the same spot each time. They can do this even in winter, when the fog gets so dense that passing vessels are detected by their wake alone and navigation is done by radar. This is a miserable time, for pilots and medical crew alike, on the icy canals in heavy snow.

Motoring down the canal San Lio and past the Cavazza Foscari we emerge just under the Rialto Bridge. Here we slow down and moor against a grand row of steps rising out of the lapping water and leading into the imposing entrance of L'Ufficio Postale, the city's post office. It may be the best access to the city's most famous bridge, but a little awkward on the way back, as patients need to be taken out through post office queues in order to reach the boat.

'Mind yourself,' says Manuela as we disembark onto algae-slathered stone. We don't want to end up in the drink. Drink, come to mention it, is quite the wrong word for the Venetian canals. Friends warned me that getting any of it in the mouth can be lethal and necessitates forty injections. Mentioning this to the head of the *ambulanza*, Dr Lodovico Pietrosanti, he laughed and said, 'Maybe not forty, but at least thirty.' Whatever the number of injections one needs, Venice is no family water park. Unlike the Hindus of India who've long immersed themselves in the holy Ganges no matter how filthy, the only Venetians found in the water are dead ones. Even now, Venetians still talk about the midnight swims taken by Lord Byron when he lived here in 1816. Almost two centuries later, just under half the buildings still remain without sewerage systems connected to the main pipes. These continue spewing their waste into the canals, and were it not for the replenishing tide, a job on the waterways of Venice would be intolerable. Despite the occasional whiff of excrement, it's difficult to resist diving from the ambulance for a cooling dip under the beating sun in summer. The only tourists seemingly oblivious to the putrid waters are those giggling Japanese girls who love nothing more than to frolic slipperless in the Piazza San Marco whenever it is flooded.

Shame it is that our pilot – an expert navigator – must remain with the boat. By the time we have walked to the end of the Calle del Galiazzo the house numbers have lost any logical progression. From what I can make out, they never had any proper sequence in the first place. Venetian addresses are generally given as one of six districts known as *sestier*, followed by house numbers. Names of the *calli* – the alleyways of Venice – are generally ignored because many share the same name. Worst of all are the haphazard house numbers, several thousand of them, frequently jumping or dropping, occasionally by more than a hundred. When this happens, ambulance crews begin a feverish hunt or return to the boat and re-evaluate. Of course there is a tatty 'canal directory' in the glovebox of the boat, but rarely does it correlate with the reality.

For a city so commonly visited and charted there seems, at any one time, to be more people wandering around lost than actually knowing where they are going. Sometimes almost everyone we pass is hunched over an expanded map, looking utterly perplexed. For those on the loose itinerary of a holiday, getting lost is part of the charm, the adventure and fun of Venice. This fun is slightly dampened for ambulance crews knowing someone's life hangs in the balance.

None of my colleagues will leave the station in Castello without consulting a giant map pasted over a wall. Getting a closer look is done with a magnifying glass the size of a dinner plate attached to the end of a rubber rope. Passionate exchanges around this map about the best access to a case often take minutes, but these discussions are never considered a waste of time. An extra minute or two planning can save an hour of wandering in circles. Venice is, after all, a labyrinth. And while some say a labyrinth's purpose is to baffle evil spirits, only fools or those without a particular objective will enter a maze without seeing it first from above.

Satellites do this best, of course, and in real time. Yet the navigation devices trialled in Venice in 2010 proved disastrous. Ambulances were sent down canals too narrow, canals with tethered boats preventing passage, canals with bridges too low and canals so shallow some boats ran aground on the way to critical cases. No one was surprised. Venice has always defied technology because technology is generally designed for a universal market and a modern world. The unique can be beautiful and confounding at the same time.

A cramped Venetian apartment built in the eighteenth century is no place to conduct resuscitation. Atmospheric golden light from a monolithic chandelier bathes the lifeless body of a man in his fifties, his gut a legacy to pasta and parmigiano, his stubbled face expressionless and grey.

Carlo, our registered nurse for the shift, takes a pulse. He knows the man's heart has stopped beating, but even doctors make mistakes. Once upon a time, in the Middle Ages, enough Venetian doctors incorrectly declared people dead that a ban was placed on burial. Those suspected of being deceased were carried to the bell towers of Venice instead and left there for weeks, just to be sure.

There is no pulse but the monitor shows what looks like a sinus rhythm. It's a confusing circumstance for junior medics – a monitor displaying normal electrical activity yet without a corresponding pulse. In these cases the heart is too damaged to respond. And while our modern day electro-cardiographs may have solved the problem of accidentally burying the living, we still can't let go.

Even thirty years back the same man at our feet without breath and without pulse would have been afforded his rightful dignity and carried to his bed, covered by a crisp white sheet, his eyes gently closed and his fingers clasped around a freshly cut rose. Now that we see a rhythm with no output, we do what paramedics and doctors do around the world. We pound up and down on his chest with CPR, popping ribs off their sternal fixtures. We insert cannulas and push in adrenalin boluses. Everyone works quietly. It's a well-rehearsed production, despite all of us knowing it's just about impossible to survive a cardiac arrest unless one collapses in the path of an ambulance.

Manuela has a difficult time with the endotracheal tube. I can see the man's mouth doesn't open much and he has a bull neck.

'His tongue,' says Manuela for my benefit, struggling to push it aside. *'Un elephante lingua!'*

She gets the tube in, but seconds after she ties it off, things become complicated.

'*Il polso, il polso!*' Carlo announces urgently, his fingers against the man's neck.

Manuela raises her eyebrows. '*Stai scherzando?*' she says, literally 'Are you kidding?'

Her expression, like everyone else's, is one of dismay rather than joy. Usually, following a few standard treatments, the patient remains dead and we leave his body to the funeral directors and their sleek water hearse. Instead, the man has gotten himself a pulse. This is the problem with adrenalin in cardiac arrest. Even a headless body, they say, can be made to appear alive with a shot of it. Adrenalin is the deliverer of false hope. Families watch and wait and imagine that death may have been nothing but a terrible dream, a slumber from which their beloved will wake at any moment.

It is clear to us all we now must load and transport the patient. For a few minutes we bumble about, moving equipment from one place to another, hoping the adrenalin will wear off. But the pulse is still there. Every one of us is looking at the man's enormous belly and estimating his colossal weight in our heads. Every one of us is picturing the journey ahead – the six flights of narrow eighteenth-century stairs we ascended in a stoop, the tourist-crowded alleyways of lumpy cobblestones, the lifting onto our dangerously swaying boat and riding the choppy lagoon to a hospital where the man will, no doubt, be 'declared dead' soon after.

At the Pronto Soccorso – the emergency room of L'Ospedale – the charismatic head of department, Dr Michele Alzetta, is unimpressed. Two weeks earlier we had taken espresso in his office and swapped stories about our respective experiences in South Africa where he'd grown up. During our discussion it became apparent Alzetta possessed an unbridled realism in respect to cardiac arrest. By transporting pulseless patients, he told me,

Anglo-American ambulance services were indulging in a sort of heroic, almost romantic, fantasy. In Venice, on the other hand, ambulances only move patients with a cardiac output.

The rationale made perfect sense to me. Be it a case of ventricular fibrillation or asystole, the patient should be treated on scene until one of two things occur. Either they regain a pulse or they do not. If their heart is started again – transport them. And if after a concerted resuscitation attempt there is no sign of life – call it quits. The Venetian conditions have played a big part in the adoption of this simple approach. Effective CPR is pretty much impossible while carrying a patient down six flights of stairs and through the congested passageways of the city. Worse is the application of chest compressions on water. It is hard enough to keep an unconscious patient from rolling off the stretcher as the flat-bottomed boats traverse the choppy lagoon. Recent studies show that continuous and effective CPR is the most important factor for positive outcomes in cardiac arrest, more so than pharmacology. Thus, Alzetta argues, if CPR cannot be effective in transit, what is the point of moving a patient who needs it? Even in a road ambulance, I tell him, with heavy braking and the mounting of median strips, I must grip a crossbar with one hand and compress the patient's chest with the other – convincing me long ago of its futility.

Then there is defibrillation. The delivering of a biphasic current through the heart to neutralise its aberrant activity and restore a functional rhythm can be dangerous for those applying it. Angelica – a close colleague of mine in Sydney – was accidentally defibrillated a few years back by her partner, a medic of Russian origin who may have mistakenly called 'Clear!' in her native tongue. Either way, Angelica was still doing CPR when the patient was zapped. And because any contact with the victim, or stretcher on which they lie, can result in the rescuer also being electrocuted, road ambulances are required to pull over and stop for the safe delivery of a shock. Due to the constant wake from other vessels, however, pulling over on the Grand Canal of Venice is problematic.

'As you well know, Benjamin, all these heroics are of little use anyway,' said Dr Alzetta before I left his office that morning. 'Resuscitation is mostly a matter of smoke in the eyes of a dead man's loved ones.'

Even after we tell Alzetta that our patient from the Calle del Galiazzo had a pulse upon loading which he promptly lost again near the Sacca della Misericordia, he is writing up the death certificate. Having worked on the ambulance boats himself, he knows as well as any of us that Manuela has continued the resuscitation in transit to avoid doing paperwork. In any case, it is universally understood that no one dies in an ambulance. People can be dead on the scene, but if loaded up they're considered alive or, at the very least, 'suspended' between life and death until they reach the hospital. Ambulance services have historically considered it bad for their reputation when the newspapers print that a patient 'died in the ambulance'. These days, public relations departments are sure to emphasise in their press releases that a patient was 'dead at the scene' or 'died soon after arrival' at the hospital. This 'dying soon after arrival' is exactly what has happened today, on the first day of summer in La Serrenissima.

Behind the department of traumatology, in ambulance service headquarters, Manuela unlaces her cherry-red Doc Martin boots, scuffed by a thousand adventures through the Venetian wilderness. She places them beside a recliner on which she leans back with a sigh and opens the first page of a novel she has taken from the station bookshelf. It is Dostoevsky's *L'eterno Marito*. Reading is her passion and her escape. From the misery of ambulance work she departs into the imaginary worlds of her favourite authors. In particular, Jewish writers Amos Oz, David Grossmann and AB Yehoshua, whom she describes as *bellissimo*! Since working with her I have noticed she begins to read at the earliest opportunity after a difficult case and doesn't stop until the next one comes along.

How cultured these Venetian medics are with their bookshelves full of classical literature! Even the tradesmen in this city who stop at bars for afternoon beverages in their dust-covered overalls will sip on wine, caring nothing for beer, as one might expect. This refined culture extends also to fashion. Dressed as they are in swish designer suits and stylish cravats, locals are easy to spot among tourists wandering about in short shorts and Hard Rock Café T-shirts. Venetians are known for their fashion sense and it's no wonder the medics of the *ambulanza* share an obvious distaste for the fluorescent orange Gore-Tex they must wear at work.

On the station meal table where ambulance crews will later spread their communal *pastasciutta*, they now take out Venetian playing cards known as *Trevigiane*. These cards first appeared in the fourteenth century and still remain in use across the Veneto region. With an appearance similar to that of tarot, they feature a series of colourful figures holding symbolic accessories. The trick-taking games using *Trevigiane* are played in teams and demand complex strategies and secret codes conveyed by means of subtle winks and raised eyebrows. Venetian medics tell me the games were passed down to them by their own fathers and there is every chance that *Scopa* and *Briscola* were played close to this spot by the original ambulance gondoliers of Napoleon's Venice.

It is the quietness of the card-playing that I find most refreshing. It's about the only time these medics stop talking. Perhaps even more so than other Italians, Venetians are famous for their multilayered, breathless conversation and apparent ability to talk and listen simultaneously.

A fax arrives at the station from the headquarters of the *carabinieri,* a notice about a missing English girl, a musician.

'They'll find her at the house of some gondolier,' jokes one of the boatmen, sparking a fit of giggles round the table.

Morale is in fine form. The staff are young, vibrant and energetic. In a corner of the station above last year's mini Christmas tree hung with now dusty baubles are photos pinned to a corkboard. There's a picture of nurse Adriano pointing at a floating fish and one of Gilberto and Luca sunbaking on the deck of an ambulance. Another shows a whole group of doctors and nurses at their annual summer party on pilot Folegatti's private launch, dressed in drag and clinking glasses of *prosecco.* The camaraderie of these men and women is unquestionable. In uniform they kiss one another tenderly on both cheeks whenever they arrive or depart from work. And although I may not qualify for kisses yet, I always get a warm smile and hearty, '*Bongiorno* Benjamino!'

Unable to play the card game, I flick through a pile of Italian emergency medical journals, looking at the pictures of semi-exposed brains and X-rays of thoraces penetrated by road signs. There is also a catalogue of rainbow-coloured stethoscopes and a signature perfume for paramedics contained in elegant glass bottles shaped like the Star of Life. More interesting are the custom ambulances for sale. One series advertised has interiors painted by artists Marian Alfredo and Figlio Pistoia, specialists in the rendering of Walt Disney dreamscapes, sunsets and happy clouds or underwater worlds of smiling mermaids and dancing seahorses. These *Bon Fanti* ambulances for neonates and children also come with plain pink or baby blue interiors. For the discerning adult patient, classic frescoes in the tradition of the Sistine Chapel are available for the ceiling of an ambulance on special request. One suggestion made by the company is Michelangelo's depiction of the Apocalypse with souls of the newly departed being judged by

Christ and his saintly entourage. As paramedics we often forget the view our patients are getting in their final moments on earth; those blank ceilings, air-conditioning vents and fluorescent lights are awfully profane. Ambulances decorated with a beautiful Renaissance fresco of heavens opening, on the other hand, though more expensive, would make a marvellous entry to eternity.

As each call comes into the station, a control tower on *terra firma* known as 'alpha uno' decides the composition of an appropriate team based on the nature of the case. Code Green cases, like the waking of a drunk, for instance, will only require the services of a pilot and a pair of operators trained in basic life support. Code Yellow cases will need at least an *infermiere*, a clinical nurse specialist, while life-threatening Code Red cases require the inclusion of the *medico*, the doctor on duty, of which there is only one available at any time. The concept of an ambulance paramedic as we know it does not exist in Italy and the word has little status. Vincenzo Nardacchione, the lab-coat-wearing medical director of the L'Ospedale Civile made this very clear to me while I sat in his office last month when he said, 'A nurse may be slave to the doctor, but a paramedic is slave to the nurse.'

Although the correct definition of the word 'paramedic' may be a medical all-rounder capable of doing a little bit of everything, in Anglo-American systems this medical all-rounder can apply complex procedures and administer drugs that most nurses are unable to outside a hospital. Nardacchione waved his hand dismissively when I told him of the reverence given to paramedics in Australia and America. Seems the traditional medical model and its hierarchy is alive and well in ancient Venice and won't be changing any time soon.

If laughter echoes through the hospital corridors it is coming most likely from the meal room of the *ambulanza* or behind the glass doors of Café Love, the hospital cafeteria, where ambulance crews frequently go for their espresso or, on summer afternoons, an ice-cream. But this joviality is left behind on the Fondamenta Nuove whenever we launch. Out in the canals and on the scene of emergencies the crews are remarkably reserved. Most people would probably consider this appropriate. But to me it's a little surprising. Ambulance medics the world over will commonly invoke at least a *little* comedy to relax and distract their patients. In Venice they are not so daring. Anna-Lisa, a bubbly nurse with a mane of wild black hair who assisted at our cardiac arrest, blames Venetian patients. They are too conservative for humour in the face of crisis, she tells me. Some would even consider it blasphemous.

'If I make a joke, the patient will say *tuio morgi cani*. In Veneziano it means I was raised by dogs.'

She rolls her eyes and shakes her hair. Sick Venetians are just no fun. Already some of the men have asked me not to write too much about *Trevigiane* in case a Venetian reader makes a complaint that ambulance staff have nothing better to do than play cards. This problem is worldwide, I tell them. If an ambulance pulls over at a coffee shop in Sydney, some good citizen will invariably cast their judgment. It's a slap in the face after putting our total physical and emotional resources on the line for the saving of lives, to then be feeling as if taking a break is shameful. How can we 'look busy' when there is no one to treat? Should we, in these quiet moments, be orchestrating some drama instead of playing cards? And what about firefighters? Should they also light up a few homes to avoid the accusation of laziness?

At least the medics here can relax behind closed doors. And now, between card games, the moon-faced pilot, Sandro del Acqua – quite the appropriate name for a boatman – amuses us with tales of his teenage antics. Most entertaining is the story of how he secretly fed laxatives to the pigeons on the Piazza San Marco which led to hundreds of unsuspecting tourists being splattered with bird shit while queuing for the basilica. Everyone likes this story. As important as tourism is to a Venetian's livelihood, including those working for the health services, tourists are still considered the equivalent of a kidney stone or severely sprained ankle.

Dr Lodovico Pietrosanti has split the shift with Manuela Silvestri. He arrives in civilian clothes – a smart lemon-yellow shirt and stylish red-framed glasses. Like Elton John, he wears a different pair of outrageous spectacles each day. Having just come from an art gallery where he had lunch, he tells the group of his surprise at how good the polenta was. This surprises me too because I've never tasted a good polenta and don't believe there is such a thing. It is, quite possibly, the most tasteless and inedible dish ever invented. The last one I had, served in classic Venetian style with squid in its black ink, was a traumatic experience I will never forget.

On my very first day in Venice I knew we'd become friends, Dr Pietrosanti and I. He is quietly spoken, self-deprecating and extremely charming. He also insisted I call him 'Lodo' and that I join him for coffee and brioche in the mornings before work. An hour after we met he took me to his office to show me one of his prized possessions – a Queensland Ambulance Service cloth patch he'd been given as a present by a fellow doctor at a medical conference on Australia's Gold Coast. Fortunately I was able to present him with a more superior Ambulance Service of New South Wales roundel, and our friendship was sealed.

It impresses me knowing the chief of the Venetian ambulance service still works on the road, or more correctly, on the water. No one could accuse this manager of being out of touch. Of course, it's easier finding time to do this when in charge of only three ambulances.

'Confetti?' he asks, as I follow him into his office. I nod and

Lodo opens a tin he keeps in his jacket, offering me one of the little white sweets. As ambulance workers across the world know, if woken for a case in the middle of the night one never has time to brush the teeth. Little mints are ideal for staying fresh. Years ago I carried a small dispenser of peppermint Tic-Tacs, but after a series of cardiac arrests I decided to give them up. It was embarrassing when during the rigorous performance of CPR, a packet of Tic-Tacs in my top pocket rattled away louder than a Cuban maraca.

Lodo is known among his staff as a great lover of gelato. Luckily, Venice has ample supply of it. Gone are the days of local butchers and bakers and candlestick-makers. Nowadays the city is all tacky tourist shops and endless *gelaterie*. Unlike his colleagues who have moved out of Venice to improve their deteriorating diet, Lodo considers it heaven. Being one of the only ambulance doctors who still lives in the city, he is able to spend his days off walking from one gelateria to another, from *campo* to *campo*, often for hours, stopping to sample the flavours on offer.

'A man who walks is a man who needs gelato,' he says. 'Some will go for a cold *granita* or a *spritz*, but I am loyal to *gelati*.'

It occurs to me that gelati may do for Lodo what great authors do for Manuela – a pure and perfect stimulation of the senses. Like an evocative story, gelati has the capacity to facilitate an escape to distant places, fantasy worlds created by myriad flavours. A recent scientific study in the United Kingdom supported this theory, concluding that flavours of ice-cream are able to elicit emotional triggers, stimulating the transporting effects of the human imagination. And so, when Lodo tastes banana gelato he is taken to Panama, with pistachio he flies to Persia. Of all the flavours available in Venice, *mandele* – the almond – is his favourite, and takes him to the heart of a Middle Eastern bazaar.

Lodo is not alone in his appreciation for ice-cream. Most ambulance workers around the world share his weakness to some degree. In fact, I have long suspected it to be a vital component of our coping mechanism. Ice-cream's ability to light up the brain's orbitofrontal cortex is already well known since the Institute of Psychiatry in London used an MRI in 2005 to scan the brains of people eating it. Such a test may be a little extravagant considering how many people around the world can't even get an MRI following a car accident. But it proved what ice-cream eaters have known all along – that it makes them happy. Gelati is therefore the perfect antidote to misery and pain, the ideal remedy for an emergency doctor in Venice, enjoyed between shifts, on shifts, or both.

Few of the other doctors, nurses or boatmen are interested in spending any more time in the city of water than absolutely necessary. This is not because they do not love Venice. They adore it. But they simply can't afford it. They can't afford to live in it or eat in it or drink in it. And from what I can gather, most of them consider it well and truly lost, like a fatally disabled ship. It's a city they feel has been taken from them, a sacred place turned trashy theme park sinking under an ever-rising sea of obnoxious visitors wearing vulgar fashions and bumbling about with little sense of the history upon which they tread or the respect it deserves. But Venice has always been up for sale, traded by the very people who now shed tears for it. Some experts estimate that in another decade or two there is unlikely to be a single Venetian left living in the city.

'Two kinds of Venetians exist,' says Lodo. 'Those who are bitter and angry and constantly annoyed, and those who walk in the past like I do, who let the history absorb into them and remain in a state of denial about the present.'

I think about this and of Lodo's tolerance of tourists. There is no *calle* or *campo* or *piazzetta* that isn't jammed with them, shuffling along. No matter the degree of denial a Venetian may wish to be in about the Disneyland their city has become, there will always be a hollering American voice nearby to snap them out of it.

A young cook has been fired from a fancy *osteria* near the Palazzo del Giglio and locked himself in the restaurant's toilet with bottles of the finest wine from the cellar. And while his boss tried in vain to break down the door, the cook drank the bottles one by one. When we finally gain access, we find him paralytic and confused and too happy for a man who has just lost his job. He immediately accepts our offer of a trip to hospital when told the *carabinieri* are on their way to apprehend him for wine robbery.

Later in the afternoon we head to a bridge not far from the apartment I share with my wife and baby in Rialto, this time for a visitor who has also had too much good Italian *vino* and decided to fall asleep on a narrow *ponte* heavy with tourist traffic. A crowd of hundreds watches our arrival. Lodo is beautifully courteous at first in his attempts to wake the man, even addressing him as *maestro*. But our patient remains stubbornly unresponsive. This provokes Lodo to do the unthinkable and he delivers a series of slaps to the patient's face. Left cheek, right cheek, left cheek, right cheek – the sound of palm against face echoes along the canals.

I'm horrified.

While painful stimuli is an important tool for the gauging of consciousness, it's supposed to be a subtle art. Experienced paramedics know what sensitive areas are best to surreptitiously squeeze. We can pinch the softest skin and dig our thumbs right in, all the while appearing to bystanders as if our hands on the patient are immaculate expressions of our tenderness and care. Even in the privacy of a darkened ambulance, slapping is unheard of and strictly forbidden. Though taken aback by Lodo's technique, it seems somehow fitting at the same time, another example of sixteenth-century Venice even its physicians cannot shake. While considered archaic by the modern observer, slapping is, in fact, one of the most effective forms of painful stimuli known. Nor is there any other method ambulance workers themselves find more appealing than this, if only they were permitted to practice it. While Lodo slaps the *maestro*, I feel as much envy as I do horror and wish he would, just once, let me have a go.

Lifting the *maestro* onto our stretcher we are mobbed by a P&O tour group unleashed from the belly of their cruise ship for the afternoon, all of them dripping in sweat and led by a female guide with a microphone fastened by some contraption at her lips, holding a lollypop with 'Group D' printed on it.

'Oh my God, Jim,' I hear an American woman in the group exclaim to her husband. 'Someone's gone down!'

'Seems kinda sick, don't he.'

'Gee, I hope he's not dead, Jim.'

'Nope, he don't look dead, Hilary. See, look there, he just moved a little.'

'Where, Jim?'

'His foot, his foot moved, Hilary.'

'Oh my, it's just like off TV, isn't it, Jim?'

Their conversation is cut short by the guide who addresses her group and waves her hand in our general direction. 'And over here, ladies and gentlemen, we can see a boat ambulance of Venice at work …' She carries on after that with trivia about the hospital islands of the Venetian lagoon once used for the incarceration of the mentally disturbed and the quarantining of those with contagious diseases. The congregation of gawking humanity thickens with every minute we stay on scene, so we load up the *maestro* as quickly as we can.

Once out on the Grand Canal the *maestro* begins to vomit and I find that all we have is a pitiful little kidney dish to catch it in. Surely seasickness is not unexpected among patients travelling on water, and yet disposable vomit bags are unavailable in our *ambulanza*. No one can tell me why. This is perhaps the only distressing aspect of my work here – a bilge of salt water and emesis sloshing about my feet. Even on land, vomit bags are valued over just about every other item of gear. Without them our job would be an intolerable mess, as it is in Venice, where twice as many people vomit on the way to hospital than do on land.

Taking a shortcut to reach the Giovanni e Paolo we come face to face with a neat formation of gondolas completely blocking the canal and filled with Japanese tourists wearing broad plastic sun-visors. On one gondola there are five Japanese all packed into a heart-shaped loveseat designed for two. Our pilot throws the boat into reverse and water churns under us. While stroking the canal and waltzing back and forth on the little strip of carpet on the stern of their boats, the gondoliers are singing 'Volare' in perfect harmony. It's a divine melody – a version by The Platters, my favourite – and if not for the relentless retching of the *maestro* in the cabin the song might have made my day.

Our pilot shakes his head and curses. Behind the singing gondoliers fifteen more are queued. Our siren yelp is largely ignored as only a few try pulling over. Unconcerned, Lodo takes the time to point out a minor canal to our left down which I can see the rear wall of a palatial home he says is owned by the celebrity Count Francesco da Mosto. The eccentric count is a household name around the world thanks to his BBC television show *Francesco's Venice* and, according to a contact I have at the consulate, is also good friends with Australian politician Malcolm Turnbull.

Before I leave for home, the nightshift throws a hospital sheet over the station dining table and lays out a plate of *prosciutto* with breadsticks of impressive diameter. I know Kass also has *prosciutto* waiting for me back at the apartment but I simply can't get enough. As the slivers of divine cured ham melt on my tongue, *infermiere* Daniele Pomiato shows me a photo on his iPhone of a child's foot traumatically amputated by a *vaporetto*. The incident occurred earlier in the week and while the toes appear intact the flesh near the ankle is folded back as neatly as the *prosciutto* on my plate. Reasserting my membership of the ambulance profession I casually place another slice in my mouth and ask him if he has a close-up.

Apart from amputations, neck-of-femur fractures sustained by old people slipping on the icy cobbles in winter are about the only other trauma seen by medics in Venice, although I did attend a man who made a decent attempt at slashing his wrists last Tuesday. Luckily, he left a trail of blood we followed through the Calle Larga like Hansel and Gretel's crumbs until we found him passed out in a pencil-thin *sotoportego*. Then, about once a year or so, a speedboat of young men poaching mussels from the *vongole* farms at night collides with a *bricolla*. As for homicide, contrary to the popular novels of Donna Leon and the work carried out by her detective Commissario Brunetti, Venice sees few murders or assaults. Perpetrators would too easily get lost or cornered in some cul-de-sac without a place to hide. Besides, everyone is so packed together here no one can do anything – even in their own homes – without a witness taking note. One doctor at the *ambulanza* – Sergio Mara – transferred to Venice precisely for this security it has to offer, escaping the Calabrian mafia after a stranger at the scene of a shooting politely mentioned how prudent it would be for him and his family if the victim he was treating 'didn't make it'.

It's a sleepy old place, Venice, and these *vaporetti* injuries are the worst a Venetian medic is likely to see. First-time visitors are always a little taken aback by just how hard the ferries slam into the pier when docking. There are no gangways and passengers must step or leap onboard while the launch is heaving like a wounded beast. Such daring is not for the faint-hearted, especially in bad weather. Children are particularly prone to plunging accidentally into the gap and having their feet crushed or torn off by the sharp edges of these *vaporetti*.

Walking back to our apartment in the Rialto is possibly the most beautiful journey home a paramedic can take anywhere in the world. A journey of tranquillity and healing through alleyways that have never heard the sound of a motor car, crossing little bridges on which old men in loose cotton shirts and bold cravats sit and paint the light of sundown shimmering on water. The canals are the colour of serpentine marble at this hour, and it's no wonder Venice is the most painted city on earth.

Each day, to and from work, I pass the front door of the house where Marco Polo lived with his family in the Corte del Milion, feeling the spirit of the past rise up through the cobbles with every step. We are staying in a museum and have made it our home. Nowadays the famous *sotoportego* in both directions is guarded at one end by Maria, an accordionist with a floppy hat who neglects her bass and chord buttons and, at the other, a silent beggar crouching on his knees in the same spot, so still he could easily be mistaken for a living statue. Already I've been here long enough to be recognised by the locals who inhabit this small part of the *siestre* – an old muppet-faced man with Liberace's wardrobe, the waiters at the Osteria Di Santa Marina and the barista at Tiziano where Kass and I go for espresso and *tramezzino*, the 1.50 euro triangular white bread sandwiches with their crusts cut off, as if made by somebody's grandmother. Wearing my orange ambulance uniform home has helped garner some credibility as a local of sorts, or at least it has conveyed that I am not a tourist. Plates of spaghetti at restaurants where staff have seen me walk by now cost us half as much as they did when we first arrived, which is still, we suspect, double what locals pay.

None of the other medics or nurses or boatmen wear their uniforms to or from work. Indeed, plenty of paramedics I've known insist on changing into civilian clothes for their journeys home. This is mostly to avoid being flagged down if they come across an accident. While some might question the ethics of a medic who is capable of driving past an accident without stopping, most of my colleagues consider it essential to walk away at the end of a shift and not be drawn into another public drama. Everyone needs to get away from work, to be off duty. It's the reason celebrities wear sunglasses and baseball caps. As much as anyone, medics need to make a clean break for home, be anonymous and normal and remove their mind from the job.

Manuela, for example, wears bright elegant dresses on her way to and from the hospital. Seeing her strut along a *fondamenta* it is quite impossible to imagine she is capable of coolly feeding a nasogastric tube into a dying patient's swollen oesophagus. For her, not wearing a uniform to work has nothing to do with avoiding patients collapsed along the way. '*Non a tutti!*' she exclaimed when I asked her about it. 'Is so people don't ask me which way to the *vaporetti*, that's all!' In uniform it would take Manuela twice as long to get to work for the number of times she would have to stop and give tourists directions.

Home cooking is the only way to afford Venice and Kass has prepared her fabulous risotto, one that could outdo the finest offered by local *osterias*. Our apartment is a cosy loft criss-crossed by ancient oak beams. Our daughter Paloma sits in her highchair happily nibbling on a soggy Italian bread stick. She watches with envy as I pour a glass of red wine. This is perhaps the only affordable luxury in Venice – Italian red wine, an exceptional bottle, which can be bought for a mere 3 euros.

I take a sip and listen to Kass tell me about her day, about the galleries she visited, the districts in which she got utterly lost and how, on a whim she went looking for house number 'one'. One, of more than six thousand, that is. And after hunting for hours she found it and took a photograph. Spurred on by this success, she then decided to look for the house numbers corresponding to the birthdates of her sisters and sisters-in-law until her feet could walk no more. All in all the day would have been perfect, she says, had she not had a mishap in the afternoon while hanging the washing out the window high over our little canal. One of her lacy bras dropped into the water below and she watched it float away. In a city where every washing line is strung between canal-facing windows, I imagine plenty of laundry has vanished in this manner.

No matter, I tell her. In the morning I will look out for it on the Grand Canal.

When Kass asks me about my day she usually prefers an answer of 'good' or 'bad' rather than gory particulars. Most ambulance medics avoid bringing their work home, choosing to leave it, like their uniform, back at the station. Home is a pure and clean and happy place that must be, at all costs, preserved. While I will gladly entertain my family with comical cases – a man with a jellybean up his nostril, for example – anything grotesque or tragic is kept from them.

Falling asleep in Venice is bliss, even in the heat of summer. Like every other island, there are few secrets in the city and with open shutters we can hear the muffled voices of others enjoying their evenings. We can hear the echo of flowing wine and laughter, the meow of cats on the rooftops. Now and then comes the ringing of church bells or the baritone *Oi!* of a gondolier's warning. It's almost as if everyone is living in the same giant house. I always sleep better like this, comforted by the company of many.

Near the *piazza*, not far from the Bridge of Sighs, a Malaysian nun on a pilgrimage has fainted from the heat. Dr Lodovico steps onto the boat and we pull out from the hospital. The sun has a vicious bite and it's only 10 am.

'This nun,' scoffs Emiliano, our pilot. 'It's 33 degrees, what does she expect in a habit?'

Sprays of water fly out as we plane along the Fondamenta Nuove and turn sharply into the Rio di Giustina. I look out for my wife's bra as we go but at this speed hold little hope. We enter a maze of canals where a succession of quaint bridges are laid before us, all topped with people who have heard our siren and are setting up their cameras for a shot. While a passing ambulance may be interesting for tourists, there are equally unusual sights from our point of view. On one bridge we pass under, a frightened little Indian man is standing alone, wearing a tight gondolier's outfit and sporting a neck brace. This confuses me at first until I see a Bollywood film crew waiting for our boat to pass, ready for another take. Suddenly the premise of the film they are making comes to me in a flash. An Indian man goes to Venice. He gets a job as a gondolier. He fails to duck under a bridge. He knocks himself out and he ends up in a neck brace. Brilliant!

Further along, reclining on another lovely *ponte,* a young model allows her hair to cascade over the edge like a waterfall of honey. A gaffer beside her is beaming reflected sunlight onto her face with a white dish, while a tanned photographer in a black T-shirt contorts himself for the best angle. Notwithstanding the unconscious nun, our pilot momentarily slows under this particular bridge, as all the ambulance pilots in Venice do under bridges with attractive women on them. Perhaps I'm a little presumptuous, but I swear the male medics and boatmen never fail to glance back at a group of girls perched on a wrought-iron bridge in the hope of peeping up their skirts. This is no surprise given the reputation of the country's prime minister. Furthermore, I'm told that Casanova is reborn in every Venetian man. Cruising around and checking out the talent is by no means unique to Italy. It is, I've observed, a common pursuit in every Western nation. There is no need to tell my Venetian friends how slowly we patrol past the beach back home, they already know: all of them watch Sky TV's regular broadcast of *Bondi Rescue*. Nurse Daniele, who is an avid viewer, laments eternally about the tragic illegality of bikinis in Venice.

Halfway to hospital with our nun on board, Dr Lodo wants a twelve-lead ECG trace and asks the pilot to pull over. Our boat is tethered to a candy-striped post but continues to pitch up and down and bang against the walls of an adjacent house whenever another launch passes by. Four times we try to capture the trace until Luca, our nurse for the day, says to the pilot, 'Are we tight in? Think we're still moving.'

'Do I look like Moses?' cries the pilot, throwing up his hands in exasperation. 'Water has been like this since the beginning of time, *signore*. It's the fault of your technology, not the water!'

By now it's so hot in the cabin Lodo opens a packet of gauze and mops his brow with it. Everyone knows in this heat the tourists will begin dropping around lunchtime and, as we give up the ECG, there's talk of an early *panini*.

Café Love is unlike any other hospital cafeteria I've seen. With its low lighting, wood-panelled walls and waitresses in little white hats, it's as atmospheric as some of the best Venetian wine bars. Here we take our espressos and salami sandwiches in expectation of a busy afternoon.

Once run by friars of the Dominican Order, the rest of the hospital is equally impressive, starting with the façade, as marvellous and grand as the greatest Venetian churches. Specialists at L'Ospedale Civile have offices detailed in gold leaf and hung with oil paintings by the likes of Domenico Tintoretto and Palma Vecchio. Furthermore, various medical departments and operating theatres are still housed in the private rooms where monks used to pray. Inscriptions above each door date back to

1557. On the morning I was issued my uniform, when I tried it on in a dim and cluttered storeroom of the hospital, I looked up in astonishment at a ceiling covered in the flushed faces of cherubs drifting through a pale sky of undulating ribbons. It was a vibrant, perfectly preserved renaissance fresco, a kind of 'preview of heaven' for those dying on the beds below. Beyond art, like the rest of Venice, the hospital was constructed with no consideration for the practicalities of the future. For example, recent delivery of an MRI necessitated the removal, stone by stone, of a 500-year-old wall in order to install it. Such difficulties have resulted in the construction of a new, soon-to-be opened hospital wing with a helipad on the roof. Since most medical departments will shift there, many of my friends suspect that moments after the last patient has left the building the ancient hospital will be turned over, like everything else, to the tourists.

While Dr Pietrosanti heads to the island of Lido for a medical retrieval, I'm dispatched with *infermiere* Daniele Pomiato to a man with kidney stones – surely one of the most painful conditions a patient may experience. While Italian nurses are able to deliver a shot of morphine, they first must phone the doctor on duty at the Pronto Soccorso and request permission. Such medical control can be a hindrance to the efficiency of care and frustrating to the nurses who are well trained and experienced enough to administer the same medications paramedics in most other countries do independently. While colleagues in the United Kingdom, Australia and South Africa have their pharmacology pre-approved, even relatively safe drugs like aspirin and Anginine, vital for the early treatment of suspected heart attacks, remain unavailable to Venetian nurses.

On this occasion we are lucky our patient is morbidly intent on experiencing pain and he writhes about in the boat like a man stricken with some exotic fever.

Daniele rolls his eyes and explains, 'The church is very important in this country. Italy is home of the Pope, remember.'

What he means to point out, less cynically, is the link between pain and shame. Because the crucified Christ suffered so much, why should *we* not suffer a little? That is the philosophy. Let us suffer in empathy for Jesus. It is no wonder Italian hospitals have the lowest morphine use in the whole of Europe.

Sedatives, on the other hand, are used in Venice with perhaps more frequency than other places, Macedonia being an exception, of course. Patients suffering a psychosis or heightened symptoms of their mental illness – even those who wouldn't normally qualify for sedation – are medicated for their own safety. Such patients are prone to unpredictable behaviour, occasionally so violent no medic is willing to subdue them. Should this happen in the canals or, worse, out on the lagoon, there is a real chance the patient will end up in the water and drown. It's the same reason why heroin overdoses in Venice are rarely treated with the reversing agent Naloxone until they reach the hospital, due to the risk of the addict waking up in the boat and jumping overboard.

Motoring to the hospital we pull up behind Lodo's launch and help them unload an intubated asthma patient who is going straight to the intensive care unit (ICU). Plenty of patients sick enough for an ET tube can bypass emergency to ICU, or if it's a confirmed myocardial infarct, immediately to the catheter lab. While the latter is becoming standard practice in Anglo-American systems, bypassing emergency and proceeding directly to the specialist departments remains another benefit of having physicians on ambulances.

Over lunch, a bespectacled *Operatore Professionale*, Claudio Scarpa, recalls the days when asthmatics in Venice were treated with nebulised red wine. 'Excellent drop this one,' I imagine him telling the patient. 'It's bound to save your life, *signore*.'

Claudio is the self-professed station historian and shows me his collection of black-and-white photographs depicting ambulance gondolas gliding elegantly along the Grand Canal in a fine December mist. Their beauty is deceptive, he says. Inside these covered boats – unbeknownst to the photographer – would likely have been a sorry huddle of cholera victims. Claudio has taken it upon himself to document the activities of the ambulance service and Venice is known to have the richest and most detailed archives in the world, some dating from the ninth century. While the city is not usually associated with efficiency, when it comes to recording events and preserving official documentation, Venetians are second to none. In fact, the Archivio di Stato, only one of many Venetian archives, holds 160 kilometres of files and documents.

Working the nightshift is Dr Alfredo Musumeci, author of a paper on the history of resuscitation in Venice, a pertinent subject for a city where people come to die. Ancient manuscripts Alfredo recently uncovered in the city's libraries and archives suggest it may have been the Venetians who pioneered the public teaching of resuscitation. Over dinner we discussed the humane societies of the late 1700s and the bizarre experiments in lifesaving that were made over the preceding centuries. These were driven by Galileo's concept of experimental proof. According to Musumeci's research, it was Paracelsus, a Swiss physician and alchemist of the sixteenth century, who first put a 'reed inside a drowned man's throat' and, as a result, discovered artificial respiration. The Dutch developed mouth-to-mouth resuscitation soon after and, while the Venetians thought this was a good idea, they considered the expired air of the rescuer polluted, prompting the use of a bellows device instead. Indeed, to this very day ambulance medics around the world still squeeze a bag filled with air to ventilate their patients.

Venice was also the first city in the world to make rescue and resuscitation part of public policy. In one of the earliest examples of placing resuscitation equipment at strategic points – much like the public access defibrillation of modern times – the Venetians put portable bellows in every church and trained young monks in their use. A cash reward of four *zecchini* was issued to those who attempted to save a person drowned in the canals by giving them bellows-to-mouth. And if a citizen did not attempt to rescue or resuscitate a victim, Venetian courts were possessed with the authority to order punishment of the 'bad Samaritan', sometimes even amputating an arm or leg of the accused. Extreme measures, but lives were saved.

Unfortunately, none of this lasted. By the nineteenth century the bellows of Venice had reached London and other European cities built on waterways, but were causing widespread pneumothoraces – or collapsed lungs – from over-enthusiastic inflation. Resuscitation went backwards from there, at least for another hundred years. The recently drowned were rolled over barrels, galloped on horses and, most alarmingly, suffered the indignity of having tobacco smoke puffed up their rectums with oriental hookah pipes.

'Nothing was the same after the French took Venice,' says Alfredo, shaking his head. This is odd considering Napoleon's field doctor Baron Dominique-Jean Larrey went on to be accredited as the inventor of the ambulance and the creator of triage.

Equally interested in the history of his profession is Venetian nurse Antonio de Pra, a tall man with bulging eyes and an eccentric demeanor who wears a conspicuous ring engraved with a Maltese Cross. Much of his own free time is devoted to first aid in his capacity as a *donato* of the Venetian Cardinal of the Grand Priore of the Knights of Saint John. While the word 'of' may never have occurred so frequently in one man's title, Antonio modestly insists he is but a pilgrim of the order with the duty to give assistance to other pilgrims. As a former long-serving member of St John Ambulance in Sydney, I'm well aware of the role St John played in spreading first aid through the world, but I've rarely been conscious of the organisation's Catholic roots. Here in Italy, however, St John is considered as much a Catholic order as a voluntary ambulance service. Its Knights of Justice take strict vows of poverty, chastity and obedience just as the monks of other orders do. Becoming a *donato* was no easy matter for Antonio de Pra either, and involved sending firm proof of his Catholicism to Rome, certified by a stamp from a bishop. Antonio now plays an important part in the annual mass and procession held in Castello at a Gothic church dedicated to St John the Baptist. Venice has historically been the headquarters of St John in northern Italy and the annual mass draws devotees from across the country. The *calli* and *campi* of Castello at least are filled with *Cav di Onore e Devovione* – Knights of Honour and Devotion – resplendent in *feruca* hats and ceremonial swords. On this day every year Antonio also gets to don his monastic scapular, embroidered with a giant Maltese Cross, draped over his shoulders like a hero's cape.

In a sense, the scapulae of St John and the orange Gore-Tex of the *ambulanza* are no different to the harlequin suits and sumptuous gowns of the carnival. Because Venetians have always delighted in dressing up, costume shops abound, not to mention the pervasive merchants of the mask. On a recent weekend, Kass took our baby Paloma and me to Atelier Nicolao, one of the city's most famous costume-makers in Cannaregio for something to do. We spent the morning trying on various bodices and tights, posing like amateur thespians in front of a giant mirror, taking photos and laughing ceaselessly. I'm the first to admit I, too, enjoy donning a costume at every opportunity. I consider it a spell of sorts under which I willingly fall, my personality adapting to match whatever character the costume evokes. For this reason

I'm convinced a uniform is as much about giving the public an impression of professionalism as it is about making a demand of the wearer to 'live into' the costume they are wearing. Ambulance uniforms and gorilla suits may be nothing alike but both elicit an almost uncontrollable response in the wearer. Dressed as a gorilla, even the least theatrical person will probably act like one. Likewise, a stiffly pressed ambulance uniform infuses the wearer with a certain aptitude and confidence they may not have otherwise had before putting it on.

Usually I only smell death in the winter. But now, after lunch at Café Love, it is in the air and unmistakable. The first tourist to drop, not far from the railway station, is a German. This is no surprise to any of us. It's the very reason I'm here, working the Venetian canals in summer when just about every patient is a tourist and just about every tourist speaks German or English and not a word of Italian, let alone Veneziano. As a German–English bilingual medic, it was naive of me to assume I'd be riding along as a mere observer.

'Benjamino!' cry the nurses whenever we get a foreigner. 'Another one!' And I find myself assessing the patient from head to toe as if I'd never left home. 'Bloody hell!' said an Australian man last week, having slipped on a spot of algae. 'You're an Aussie? I can't believe it! What d'ya think of this damn ankle, mate?'

In contrast to many of their visitors, Venetians are a fit bunch. They walk the canals all year round without aid of car or scooter or pushbike. Up and down the stairs of Byzantine buildings they go, unaccustomed to elevators. The cardiovascular systems of middle-aged Venetians are, for the most part, in reasonably good shape. Some visitors, on the other hand, are so obese they're unable to pass through the narrower alleyways. Many have never walked so much in their lives. Hearts give out if pushed too far – and Venice knows how to push.

When we reach the location there is one man doing CPR and at least three hundred people standing round watching and pointing and shaking their heads. We barge our way through the crowd calling *'Permesso! Attenzione!'* and knock people aside with our gear.

Cameras flash everywhere. Above us, on the balcony of some hotel, a man leans over with a long lens, an ordinary tourist perhaps feeling for a moment like a war correspondent or daring *paparazzo*. Dozens of other onlookers also have their camera-phones out. Others take videos, as if we are no different from the jumping dolphins of a water park. There are toddlers on the shoulders of parents, geriatrics with walking sticks, a gaggle of Japanese. Yet it's no attraction to see a man, half grey, half blue, with a gaping mouth of foam and a jiggling gut, whose chest is aggressively pummelled by medics, and who, only moments earlier was haggling over some tacky souvenir that is thoroughly useless in the afterlife.

We defibrillate the German and his arms fling up with the shock, giving the crowd a final wave. The sound of three hundred people gasping at once is awesome to behold and leaves a moment of silence in which all we hear is the quiet whimpering of a frightened child. On our monitor, the German's rhythm remains in asystole – unwavering and final. It's what we're expecting and, after fifteen minutes flushing through our routine drugs, everyone agrees to stop. Reversing a flatline is near impossible. Although the German's body is in public view, we leave him there for the police launch, covered by a sheet, the closing curtain at the end of our show. An officer of the *carabinieri* will find the man's hotel and inform his wife or tour group.

Anecdotally – according to my colleagues at least – the majority of visitors who die in Venice are Germans. Manuela for one is convinced that Germans consider it as sacred to die in Venice as Hindus consider it to die in Varanasi. A logical explanation of this would be the popularity of the destination among retired Germans. But I also find it an unusual coincidence that Wagner, one of Germany's greatest composers, also died in the city, as did Gustav von Aschenbach, the protagonist of Thomas Mann's book *Death in Venice,* a celebrated piece of German literature about a man's last days in the city.

Venice has long been associated with death and Germans have no monopoly on dying here. The city is widely known as one of shadow and decay. Each morning on my way to work I watch funeral boats departing from the Fondamenta dei Mendicanti for the nearby cemetery island of San Michele or the airport for expatriation, their shiny black coffins draped with flowers. Records show that Venice has, over time, endured more than seventy visitations of the plague. One of these, in 1575, wiped out a third of the population and the canals were crammed with floating corpses. Back then it was also a city of night-time assassinations and public hangings. In his book on Venice, celebrated historian Peter Ackroyd describes its waters as the 'emblem of oblivion'. There is, indeed, something consoling about death near water. It would certainly be a romantic way of dying, if dying can be described as romantic. Poet Robert Browning died here and Lord Byron, the greatest of romantics, had every intention to, from the moment he arrived.

We are packing up our gear when Claudio mentions he will be checking YouTube later in the evening to see if we've been uploaded. Doing this has become the habit of many Venetian medics – scouring the web for videos in which they appear and it's not because they want to be famous. I'm told that many clips have been reported and deleted through respect for patients' privacy. I suspect the real reason has more to do with Venetian medics not wanting their patient care scrutinised. Manuela admits to me in private her greatest concern about getting on film is the possible millions who may see her lying gracelessly in a puddle of canal water, tubing a patient. Whenever I work with the diva I catch her angrily scolding tourists with their cameras out, *'No! No! No permesso! Pazienza!'* Once, while busy taking the blood pressure of a woman collapsed in the Rialto, a male tourist was foolish enough to tap her on the shoulder and ask if she could pose with him in a photo. This is not uncommon. Another *medico* had the same thing happen to him a month ago while struggling to stop a patient having a seizure on the cobbles. What both of these incidences confirm is a belief held by many visitors that Venice is somehow unreal, like an interactive theme park. Instead of Mickey Mouse and Donald Duck, tourists in Venice get to see a boat ambulance in action. Can they really be blamed for this? What the *ambulanza* offers is a refreshing change from the cold statues and motionless façades of the past.

Who expects privacy in Venice anyway? Nowhere is safe. Venetian society has historically been one of spectacle, of events and celebrations to draw the visitor and impress foreign dignitaries. While the city is known for its annual carnival, the biennale and its film festival, it has always been famous for public entertainment in the form of outdoor theatre, elaborate fetes, wild beast shows and pyrotechnics occurring at many times of the year. During the Austrian bombardment of Venice in 1848, locals watched the action from their balconies with opera glasses. Many earlier examples of morbid curiosity existed in Venice too, such as mock funeral processions in the 1700s and disfigured individuals being pushed around in barrows for public amusement. Now, as our ambulance trolley clatters over the cobbles and multitudes stop to watch us go by, little has changed. Henry James once described Venetians as 'members of an endless dramatic troupe'. And a troupe is what I feel I've joined.

As Murphy's Law dictates, the instant I receive a cold can from the hospital's *chinotto* machine another call comes in. Temperatures have reached 40 degrees and an older British woman has collapsed near San Martino. Even with assistance she is unable to get up. On closer examination, Lodo suspects she has a fractured neck-of-femur. It's just before three in the afternoon and her cruise ship is due to depart for Greece at four. This is the time most liners leave the Venetian lagoon in one slow and splendid convoy. Her holiday has ended before it has even begun. Her belongings will be delivered to the hospital and she will soon be on a flight back to England for surgery.

Our next case involves a difficult extrication from the top floor of a building with a narrow staircase. Claudio and a female BLS medic by the name of Betty Busetto carry the patient down, just the two of them lugging this ancient, red wooden chair that resembles a wheelbarrow, the only carry-chair sturdy enough to withstand lengthy journeys through the Venetian alleyways. All the way down our patient yells 'Mamma mia!' at the top of her lungs, trying her best to grab the rails and unbalance her bearers. Claudio and Betty, however, are built like Titans and hold firm. Nevertheless, back injuries are common here. Getting a patient out of an apartment is only the first challenge. Lifting a patient onto a pitching boat is just as risky. Once again there is no gangway as the relative movement of the boat against the docking point would make it dangerously unstable. Ironically, the Venetian state once contributed to the development of hydraulic technology, yet while this has been discussed a great deal, ambulance boats are simply too small to accommodate hydraulics. As for larger, wider boats, they would limit access to parts of the city already hard to reach. It is unlikely hydraulic arms would fit under the low Venetian bridges anyway.

While the ambulance is cleaned and the crew takes a short rest, Dr Lodovico insists on giving me a slideshow of photographs from his recent holiday in Las Vegas. Bizarrely, the doctor mainly went there to see 'The Venetian' casino, a re-creation, no less, of his home city, complete with a smaller version of St Mark's Square, the Rialto Bridge, towers, *calli* and canals. I can't stop smiling at the thought of a man from Venice visiting Vegas to see a fake Venice while people from Vegas visit Venice to see the real thing.

'It's my observation that the gondolas in Vegas are imperfect,' he says in a scientific tone. 'They are wider and rounder in the middle.' He points to a photo of a teenager with acne employed as a gondolier for the summer, struggling to maintain his balance with a full load. At least capsizing on the canals of Vegas wouldn't be so bad, given the purity of the casino's chlorinated waters.

Soccer fever has gripped Europe and the ambulance crews of Venice cram around the small television set, attempting to catch a little of Italy versus Slovakia between calls. All the while they lament the abysmal performance of the Italian team. How I pity the sick or injured who interrupt a sporting match, no matter how bad the home team is playing. The same can be said for rugby or horseracing in Sydney.

Pilot Luciano Nicolai gets a message on his phone. It's from the Magistrato Alle Acque – the Venice Water Authority – warning of a high tide known here as *acqua alta* expected to peak in the next hour or so. In winter months, when African winds blow up from the Adriatic, water levels can rise so high that entire districts are submerged and a warning alarm is sounded throughout the city. Moderate warnings only come via text message and these are fairly regular. Luciano closes his phone, unconcerned. Most pilots already know the bridges under which ambulances cannot pass at high tide.

Slovakia scores again and everyone swears.

Seconds later the phone rings.

Probably good timing, I think to myself. None of the ambulance crews are interested in watching Italy being massacred by Slovakia and everyone volunteers for the case simultaneously. It's a life-threatening *rosso* call. Daniele and Luciano kit up and someone knocks on Lodo's office door. In less than a minute we are skipping across the choppy lagoon with our siren blaring.

Information on the case gives every indication of another cardiac arrest. Despite this Luciano takes it easy through the Rio dei Mendicanti, especially on entering the canal San Marina. 'Wife hysterical', 'CPR in progress', 'caller panicking' – snippets of information from the scene normally make me put my foot down. But only a fool would do this in a boat without a keel.

As Luciano approaches the canal into which he wants to turn he underestimates the tidal current behind us and overshoots the mark. It happens to the best of them, but is still an embarrassment. No pilot wants to sit in a canal sideways blocking traffic, attempting to make a ten-point turn by bumping back and forth into opposing walls, especially when heading to a cardiac arrest.

Once free of the watery intersection, all of us, including the doctor, have donned our rubber gloves and don't expect another hold-up. But it's not Luciano's day. In the next canal we come up against a low bridge and scrape to a halt halfway under it. Everyone stays calm, which is commendable considering we are well and truly trapped while the patient across town remains unconscious. The crew reaches up to the underside of the bridge and tries with their hands to physically push the boat through. Inch by inch we move, to the sound of steel against stone. Finally we make it out the other side.

I begin to wonder what will happen if the tide continues to rise, blocking our return journey. It wouldn't be the first time a loaded ambulance has found itself boxed in by impassable bridges on both ends of a canal during high tide. The only options are to wait for the tide to retreat or walk to hospital. During *acqua alta alta,* an ultra high tide, the boats are only able to move through a handful of major canals, the rest of the journey completed by the crew on foot, sometimes in waist-deep water. In the winter of 2009, the tide peaked at 1.62 metres above sea level and *infermiere* Adriano Zulian waded for thirty-five minutes to reach a patient. For such a scenario each ambulance is stocked with crotch-high gumboots like the ones worn by fly-fishermen. Tales of medics forced to carry their patients slung over the shoulder through flooded alleyways for an hour back to the boat have me vow to never again complain about lifting a patient down a handful of steps. Daniele mentions that the service could well do with some rescue surfboards as used by Australian lifeguards. Only these, he says, 'will get us under the Pasqualigo Ponte'.

Helicopter evacuations are out of the question, too. Helicopter flights over Venice itself are banned for fear the city would collapse in the downdraft of rotors. Thus it remains that it is the ambulance boatmen, as much as the doctors and nurses, on whom a patient's life depends.

Giant underwater dams are currently being built at the entrance to the lagoon, designed to be mechanically elevated during *acqua alta.* Until this system is completed, however, high tide is a disastrous time of day to have a heart attack in Venice.

The next bridge we go under is as low as the last and I remember it well, having hit my head on it a few days ago. We were loaded at the time with a semiconscious patient suffering acute peritonitis when the stern drifted back and I cracked my skull against the keystone. Others in the crew recount similar minor knocks to the head from bridges, usually, they admit, in the process of inspecting an attractive *belladonna* on the *fondamenti.* Only one ambulance pilot was ever knocked out cold, while urban legend has it that a Venetian fireman once lost his entire head.

It's been at least ten minutes from the time we departed and I've seldom had such a convoluted and adventurous response to an emergency. The small canal closest to the address happens to be one we are unable to navigate, this time not for reasons of high water but because it is far too shallow. At low tide the canal is less than a foot deep. While ambulance boats have flat bottoms for exactly this reason, our pilot estimates that even now at high tide the depth is unlikely to be greater than 80 centimetres, making our passage impossible. Shallow canals like this one are why the Venetian fire brigade has mini hovercrafts at their service and the police are trialling jet skis.

'From here we walk,' says Adriano, lassoing a rope around the stone upright of an iron fence erected along a narrow path to prevent people from slipping on ice and falling into the canals during winter. I hoist our Lifepak up to Adriano and clamber over, dreading the thought of lifting an unconscious patient over a fence and into the boat. As if reading my mind Adriano says, 'This patient will not go anywhere.' Adriano has been around long enough to know. In Venice, the more difficult a time we have *getting* to a scene, the less likely it is we'll want to take the patient *out*. In the case of a dismal egress, having a doctor onboard is quite an advantage. Medical practitioners have an absolute personal responsibility for clinical judgment, a level of autonomy that paramedics and nurses are yet to achieve fully, allowing them more confidence in deciding to leave sick people at home with treatment and advice.

The seventy-eight-year-old woman is supine in bed, unconscious, with laboured breathing. Her lungs are so full of fluid we hear a rasping gurgle with every intake of breath. She is terminally ill, the family explain to us. Some would ask why, when a patient is terminal, there is a need for an emergency ambulance. Lodo thinks differently. As Adriano sets up the oxygen and I stick on some monitor dots, Lodo opens his tube kit, and slowly, methodically, without saying a word, locks blade to handle and slides it into the woman's open mouth. A glimmer of torchlight bounces back against the doctor's steady eye. A former anaesthetist, Lodo feeds the tube into her trachea with such ease he could be doing it in his sleep.

Is this a lifesaving action?

Perhaps if coupled with drug therapy and an exit strategy, it might be thought so. But the whole crew looks dug in. Adriano has pulled up a sofa beside the bed and Lodo eases himself onto the corner of the mattress, squeezing the oxygen bag whenever the woman attempts a breath. Rapid bleeping on the monitor indicates an escalating heart rate. Her body is feebly trying to compensate for total shutdown. Everyone knows the patient will soon be dead, be it here or the hospital. Better here. Not because our boat is moored 200 metres away, or that we're up six flights of uneven stairs, or because the tide is still so high. Better here because this is her home, it is where she was born, where she grew to be an adult and where she gave birth to three boys. Better here because this is where her own mother died and her mother before her.

All of her children are gone now, like most of the young of Venice who have left to start an easier, more affordable life on mainland Italy. One-third of the population is over the age of sixty and the death rate in Venice has overtaken the birth rate by a factor of four.

High up in lonely rooms like this, other old Venetians also wait to die, listening to the chatter of tour groups below with their shutters closed. Foreign romantics do not own death in Venice. Venetians do. Unlike German tourists though, Venetians die in private, and Dr Lodovico Pietrosanti is happy to allow it.

When the old lady takes her final breath it sounds as if she's inhaling under water. For a moment the thought of this unsettles me – drowning in a city that barely manages to keep its own head above water.

We switch off the machine, look at our watches and gather our disposables. It's the fifth cardiac arrest in as many days and my clothes are beginning to smell of death – of death and the sea.

No one says a word until Lodo breaks the silence. Pulling off his slippery gloves he turns and with profound gravity makes a request none of us can possibly refuse.

'Amici, un gelato?'

A HULA SAVED MY LIFE

Hawaii

Her name is Leilani, our hula girl mascot, clutching a little ukulele and wiggling her hips madly on the dashboard of the Ford. The faster we go, the faster she dances. And the faster she dances, the faster we go.

Down in Waikiki, at a high-rise apartment block sprouting from a palm grove, a local Hawaiian woman is unable to wake her husband. When the doors of the elevator open on the thirteenth floor we hear her screaming. Her pet parrot is screaming too, a rainbow toucan in a domed cage, hanging beside the sofa on which the patient is slumped unconscious and drooling.

'How long has he been like this, Ma'am?' asks Tippy Lee, a paramedic with the Honolulu Emergency Medical Services (EMS). Neither he nor his partner Chad stop to wait for an answer. Paramedics, like emergency doctors and nurses, are adept at firing off questions and rapidly acquiring a history while working on the patient at the same time.

'He just went like this suddenly now!' cries the woman hysterically.

'*Kwaark!*' screeches the toucan for emphasis, right in Tippy's ear. Tippy and Chad have the man on the carpet now, an airway in situ, bag-mask held in place for 100% oxygen, his shirt torn open and defib pads slapped on.

'Weak and slow carotid,' says Tippy. 'Regular respirations present.'

'He's in a third degree at twenty,' comments Chad.

Tippy shakes his head.

'Right, let's switch to pacing.'

'*Kwaark! Kwaark!*' cries the parrot again.

The man's heart has failed. His pulse is less than twenty now, too slow to produce enough perfusion pressure for delivery of oxygen to vital organs. Both paramedics work quickly, expertly. While Tippy ventilates, Chad pushes buttons on the *Lifepak* and dials external pacing. He selects the joules and, in order to speed up the man's heart, begins small biphasic shocks at a rate of seventy per minute, forcing the heart to contract correspondingly and increase blood pressure. As oxygenated blood works its way back around the man's brain, he begins to wake, alarmed at the regular electric charges contracting his body with a violent twitching. He tries protesting, but every shock jolts him into a stunned silence. Chad takes over ventilations now while Tippy secures an IV. After two increments of Atropine, Tippy sets up a Dopamine drip running at 10mcgs/kg/min. Seeing the patient's obvious discomfort, Tippy draws up a sedative, pushing it rapidly into the IV port.

'Sir, I'm sorry, you're heart is beating too slowly. You're receiving some electrical impulses from our machine. I know it's uncomfortable, but we're trying to keep you alive.' He then goes on to explain the effects of the medication, that soon he may feel sleepy, but more relaxed. The fire department guys come through the door as backup to help us with lifting and carrying the patient out.

'Anything we can do?' asks the fire chief, just as the parrot has another fit.

'*Kwaark! Kwaark! Kwaark!*'

'Sure,' says Chad. 'Can someone shoot that damn parrot?'

While shooting parrots is not a usual skill of the Hawaiian paramedic, shooting a 200-pound Ahi fish at sea is another matter.

Returning to the station from Queens Medical Centre we swing by Magic Island, a tropical peninsula on the edge of a beach popular among locals, well away from the holidaying hordes at Waikiki. Other ambulance crews are parked here too where they sip iced coffees between cases in a quiet and scenic spot. Tippy's other paramedic partner Mitch is among them, a muscular native Hawaiian covered in Polynesian tattoos.

'Hey Mitch, I stopped by the gun shop the other day,' says Tippy with a squeak, his voice naturally high in pitch, or as he puts it, 'like a Wahini'.

'Anything catch your eye?' asks Mitch.

'Yeah, a nice .357 Magnum, better revolver than my last one. My paramedic trainer Ben Kojima told me it's the only way to settle a big fish on the lure, beats hitting it over the head. You just reel it close enough to get a shot in, then *Bam! Bam! Bam!*

That's it. Nothing competes with a Magnum.'

'So long as you don't put a hole in your boat,' says Mitch with a chuckle.

It's the first I've heard of fish shooting, and it's not something I would have expected from Tippy Lee, the born-again Christian, surfing lover of God's almighty marine life, His creatures great and small.

In the distance, past the paddleboards and canoes, the distinctive shape of Diamond Head cranes into the sea, adorned with waving palms. We sit blinded by the flickering sunlight on water and listen to Tippy's testament. Not that he would normally offer it. But I've asked him about his faith as I'm curious how it's helped him become the paramedic he is, among the most liked and respected on Oahu.

It was beside a lake one night, during his EMT course, that Tippy came to Christ after quietly challenging God for a sign to prove his existence.

'Suddenly there was a shooting star, turquoise and so bright, much brighter than any shooting star I'd ever seen. After that there was another and another and another, until the whole sky was full of these amazing shooting stars, as if God was painting with light.'

Since then, Tippy rarely forgets to pray for his patients, usually in silence.

'I don't really know what happens, but I feel a deep sense of peace and I hope that those I've prayed for feel it as well,' says Tippy. 'Often when we pick up a homeless person or a drug addict, I ask myself how I am any different from those people in God's eyes. Knowing that God loves that person, a person who may not even believe in him, knowing that He loves and wants to help that person just as much as He wants to help me is humbling. It helps me to really care for the person more, because I can see them on an equal level, versus someone who is below me.'

I'm impressed that Tippy doesn't seem shy talking about his faith in front of work colleagues. No one takes their eyes off the surf or looks his way. That is until he says, 'And Jesus helps me intubate.'

Mitch chuckles cynically nearby. 'Holy cricoid!' he retorts, referring to the pressure normally exerted by an ambulance partner over the cricoid cartilage of a patient to assist visualization of the vocal cords.

'Funny, Mitch,' says Tippy. 'No, really, when I'm putting in the tube I ask "Please God" and whenever I do this I'll get the tube. Explain that.'

Before work, I had met Tippy at a Starbucks on Kanaina Avenue for an early bible study. He arrived in flannelette shirt, board-shorts and flip-flops. Even with Mozart playing, it was still Starbucks, still mediocre coffee. We both ordered cups of hot water as Tippy had brought along his own teabags of Irish Breakfast. I wrote my notes in silence, watching my friend meditate on various biblical passages. At one point I interrupted him, curious to know which verses most inspired his work as a paramedic.

'Matthew 25:34-40 is my favourite,' he replied without a second thought. 'What you do for the least of these people, you do for me, says the Lord.'

It is the prime motivational philosophy of the most committed religious medics and rescuers I know; be they Christian, Muslim or Jew. And like my Pakistani friends, Tippy is just as sincere in his compassion and devotion to the job. That said, his jokes are outrageous and he doesn't always play by the rules. All week, between emergency cases, this God-fearing Robin Hood has smuggled free hospital sandwiches and cans of Sprite into his ambulance, delivering them around town to homeless men and women, most of whom he knows by name. To Tippy, each one is Jesus, no matter how bad they smell.

The next morning Tippy has been teamed up with Mitch. I join them at Waikiki's ambulance station, which is little more than a small backroom of the Honolulu Fire Department's building known as Pawaa. The roof of the building is tall and thatched in traditional Hawaiian style, the grounds on which it lies planted with lush tropical flora. Tippy reverses into a parking spot with a couple of surfboards on the back of his pick-up. If we finish on time and the swell is still decent, all three of us will head out to surf. It's a tough life for Hawaiian paramedics.

Earlier in the week, EMS Chief Patty Dukes – who insisted the Mayor of Honolulu sign off on my visit – invited me to a special ceremony that will take place later in the afternoon at the edge of Lagoon Drive, not far from the airport. The ambulance service chaplain will also be there, as will District Officer Richard Kahuna, with whom I attended a trauma recently on the Likelike Highway where a trigger-happy sheriff shot a fugitive in the buttocks. Neither Patty, nor the ambulance team I'm assigned to work with, are willing to elaborate on the ceremony ahead of time, although I do hear Tippy refer to the event as a 'ritual', which serves only to deepen the mystery further.

'Let's pray we'll get there,' says Tippy. After yesterday's conversation I know he doesn't mean this figuratively.

'How was your spiritual tea this morning?' Mitch asks Tippy with just a little playful ridicule.

'Excellent thanks Mitch, and your Kava?' Tippy fires back.

Mitch smiles. 'Just fine, thanks.'

'You know Mitch, Trader Joes does eighty teabags for two dollars.'

'Two dollars? Unbelievable.'

'You can't get Irish Breakfast, though. My sister brings me boxes of it from the mainland. But Trader Joes has plenty of other teas. I'm telling you, Mitch, everything goes cheap there.'

'Kava?'

'Especially Kava.'

The control room radios in and dispatches us to a job on Kuhio Avenue in the heart of Waikiki's hotel district – a patient with a decreased consciousness. This can be due to any number of causes, ranging from strokes and overdoses, to heart attacks and head injuries. It's a common call, but paramedics don't take any chances, and Mitch pushes both sirens at once. Yes, two of them, winding up and down at separate pitches. Only in America, I tell myself, would an ambulance have more than one siren. I'm constantly looking over my shoulder, squinting into the side mirror, thinking we're being followed by another ambulance. The sound is piercing and completely unnecessary. No wonder tourists and locals alike plug their ears with their fingers whenever an ambulance screams through Waikiki, shattering the quiet holiday atmosphere. People plugging their ears in Australia are considered wimps and objects of paramedics' constant amusement. But here the siren is a real health risk. Even Tippy wears industrial earmuffs, like giant headphones, whenever we're heading to a call. Just yesterday, when a member of the public dialled 911 after developing a ringing in his ear, Mitch didn't hesitate to dryly remark that, 'We've all got ringing in the ears, buddy.'

The Honolulu Fire Department has beaten us to the job once again. Tippy manoeuvres our mammoth ambulance around the yellow tiller fire truck measuring 55-feet long, taking up the entire street. I notice a Malibu surfboard hooked to the side of the ladder unit, printed with the word RESCUE. Eight firemen in fluorescent jackets stand about directing traffic and diverting pedestrians around the incident.

All this for a woman 'feeling tired'.

'How long have you felt tired for?' asks Tippy earnestly.

'The whole week,' says the woman.

'Oh dear,' says Tippy.

And we watch as the woman gives us a demonstration of being tired by nodding off, her head dropping down and up again.

'See,' she says. 'Can't stay awake.'

There are plenty of calls like this in Hawaii. People tired, intoxicated, anxious, lonely, hearing voices, depressed. How can it be, that one is depressed in this sun-drenched idyll? Tippy's theory is that some visitors are making a futile attempt to physically escape unhappiness back home, without realising their unhappiness lies within themselves and accompanies them wherever they go. But by far the most numerous of these customers are homeless men and women, many suffering addictions or mental health disorders, or both. Some are native Hawaiians affected by the recent downturn in the economy, others unemployed Micronesians. But the vast majority of homeless hark from mainland U.S.A.

After putting the tired woman to bed at Kapi'olani Medical Centre, we swing by the end of Ward Avenue where hundreds of homeless have pitched tents between palm trees near the harbour.

'This is nothing compared with Waianae,' says Mitch, referring to an area on the leeward side of the island. 'Up there it's a tent city far as the eye can see.'

'What about public housing?' I ask.

'Unless you're a Melanesian from Bikini Atoll where we tested our mushroom cloud, you don't get a house in Hawaii.'

Visiting Oahu, it's hard to miss the homeless who shuffle through Waikiki in staggering numbers, many black with dirt, hair mattered and clothing torn, pushing shopping trolleys of belongings past tourists in Aloha shirts sipping cocktails at bamboo bars. Almost every park bench all along Kalakaua accommodates a tramp or two, begging off passing tourists. Once they have enough money, Mitch tells me, many purchase a US$12 flagon of wine, drink it up and collapse on the main drag. That's when people call 911.

While official figures put the number of homeless at around seven thousand, local paramedics believe it may be as high as nine or ten thousand, quite a number for an island to accommodate.

'Being a paramedic in Hawaii was one of the best jobs in the world until the Mayor of New York gave hundreds of homeless people free one-way tickets to Honolulu,' says Mitch. 'We only know this because so many homeless we pick up in the ambulance tell us the same story.'

'It wasn't just New York,' adds Tippy. 'San Francisco and

Detroit did it too. For a person sleeping rough it might sound like a good deal, you know, the warm weather all year round.'

'And the holiday dollar,' says Mitch.

'Yeah, people on vacation give more to beggars,' says Tippy. 'But employment opportunities here are limited, and the cost of living and housing is much higher than on the mainland. Also, we don't have the same mental health facilities like other states do.'

Ironically, homelessness in Hawaii has become so pervasive that the government of the archipelago is considering legislation to give homeless people originating from other states one-way tickets out again. Plane rides back to New York would cost Hawaii about US$350 each; much less than the estimated US$35,000 per person per year it costs to provide them with ambulances, hospital care and other public services. Absurd as it sounds, if this bill is passed, those living on the streets of certain U.S. cities could theoretically take any number of round-trip holidays to Hawaii every year without paying a single dime.

While we wait for three paper cones of flavoured shave-ice, Tippy takes a call from Patty Dukes. Everything has been arranged for this afternoon's event. Again I try and extract details from Tippy about the so-called 'ritual', but he won't elaborate.

'You'll see,' he says, winking at Mitch.

The last special occasion arranged by Patty Dukes was a live demonstration of the Honolulu EMS cardio-pulmonary resuscitation education program, the original reason for my visit. Hawaii happens to be one of the most successful American states in educating the public in resuscitation, and I'd heard about the novel way in which they had achieved this.

It was called the 'CPR Hula'.

Unlike anything I'd come across before, paramedics in uniform festooned with purple leis danced a specially choreographed hula for me on the edge of a secluded beach, their hands moving in a well-rehearsed series of actions mimicking the head tilt, mouth-to-mouth and chest compressions of CPR. Beside them, a band of native Hawaiian paramedics played guitars and sung in harmony.

> *Ka'a Malama Ola says to you,*
> *'Learn CPR, it's not hard to do.*
> *Come do the CPR Hula with me,*
> *and you can help your family.'*
>
> *If someone goes down, shake him and shout,*
> *'Are you okay, bruddah, or are you knock out?'*
> *If he neva answer, don't hesitate.*
> *Call 911 'cause you no can wait.*
>
> *Chorus:*
> *Minutes seem like hours, but you're not alone,*
> *Ka'a Malama Ola is rolling to your home.*
> *Listen to the folks at 911,*
> *They're here to help you help your loved ones.*

And so it went, while Chief Dukes, creator and lyricist of the song, acted out the scenario on a Resusci Anne, her lei occasionally getting in the way of her compressions. 'Ka'a Malama Ola', she explained later, is the Hawaiian word for ambulance.

> *Feel the pulse – Auwe No Mo!*
> *Get ready to pump, don't run for the door.*
> *Bare the chest and find your place.*
> *Don't worry bruddah, we'll set the pace.*
>
> *Chorus:*
> *Minutes seem like hours, but you're not alone,*
> *Ka'a Malama Ola is rolling to your home.*

Listen to the folks at 911,
They're here to help you help your loved ones.

Pump one, two and three and four.
You're doing great, lets pump some more.
Fifteen times will help your friend.
Watch your elbows, don't let them bend.

Chorus:
Minutes seem like hours, but you're not alone,
Ka'a Malama Ola is rolling to your home.
Listen to the folks at 911,
They're here to help you help your loved ones.

They may have a song and dance about resuscitation, but I haven't worked a single cardiac arrest – or 'code' – since arriving in Hawaii. Instead it's all heat rash, sunburn and sore feet. To each of these we go with lights and sirens, the siren even at night, even through empty streets. Stable patients get the siren too, all the way to hospital.

It's the rules, they tell me, even without much traffic.

Problem with having a double siren sounding relentlessly is the attention it attracts. While a siren is designed to alert other road users to an approaching emergency vehicle, it also alerts those feeling a little unwell to a notion they may not have otherwise been entertaining in that moment. 'Ah!' they think as their ears prick up to the sounding wail, 'Now *that's* what I need! An ambulance!' Why else would we so frequently be called to cases, consecutively, in the very same street? Happens worldwide, but most commonly, I propose, in countries where the siren rings right to the doorstep. Last week, on night duty, one patient even admitted to it. Said he was feeling depressed, heard the ambulance siren, thought he deserved one too, and called 911. After hanging up he got to thinking we might be unimpressed with him unless he made some attempt at harming himself. So he put a plastic bag over his head – only for half-a-minute or so – knowing by law we'd have to take him to hospital, which we did. Had he not heard the siren in the first place, he may have just gone to bed and visited his therapist in the morning.

There's a patient with a headache on Olohana. Mitch drives this time and our hula girl is excited. Again the street is filled with firemen and fire trucks with beacons still flashing. Unlike ambulance services across most of the U.S.A., the Honolulu EMS is not partnered with the fire department. Although this is about to change, paramedic services remain separate. Even so, the fire department has for a long time been dispatched to most cases, often beating the ambulance by a couple of minutes at best. It seems an expensive enterprise, running an ambulance *and* a ladder truck to every intoxicated patient or person with indigestion. I wonder aloud if oxygen applied a few minutes early really makes that much of a difference in the majority of cases. Probably not, my colleagues agree. But it's worth it for that occasional cardiac arrest, to apply the earliest defibrillation. It's also worth it for the lifting. Back in Sydney, my ambulance partner and I carry our patients down flights of stairs. Here, the firemen do it. My friends cynically suggest too that this 'double response' conveniently inflates fire department statistics and ultimately boosts their annual budget.

'They already get way more money than EMS,' says Mitch.

Back in the east area of Sydney where I work, many of our patients call us for emotional disorders, depression and loneliness. The last thing a suicidal person wants is a fire truck arriving in their street like the Starship Enterprise unleashing a squad of burly, helmeted men marching into their bedrooms.

'What about psychiatric cases?' I ask Mitch.

'Even a fireman knows how to hold a hand,' he replies.

*

We shelter from a tropical rain shower at the Diamond Head diner and decide to get lunch while we're there. I order a Teriyaki burger, reminded of the Japanese influence in Hawaii once again. Many of the state's paramedics are of Japanese descent and the place is full of Sushi bars. There's even a six-foot Hello Kitty on Kuhio wearing a grass skirt and lei.

'Well, I think it's time,' says Tippy as we finish our lunch and the shower clears. Mitch slurps up the rest of his soda and gets up. Soon we're on the highway out of Waikiki, heading in the direction of the airport. Our radio, quiet until now, begins lighting up with jobs, some in our area.

'All covered,' Mitch reassures me. 'We're off-line, expected at the ritual.'

When we reach the turn-off to Lagoon Drive, Tippy and Mitch have become quiet. Then, a little further on, Mitch says, 'Up ahead, Tippy, on the left.'

Peering through the front window from the back cabin I can see a group of EMS vehicles parked on a strip of grass between the road and the bay. Tall snaking palms wave in a breeze high above them.

We park beside another ambulance and I let myself out the side door. For a second I'm blinded by flashes of sunlight off the water. When my eyes adjust to the glare I find myself assembled with a group of paramedics. Each one stands with their hands neatly folded in front of them. A woman comes by and tenderly places a lei of frangipani over my head. Off to the left, in the shadow of an ambulance, Chief Patty Dukes oversees proceedings.

Suddenly, from behind the slender trunk of a palm tree, a man in paramedic uniform buttoned all the way up steps out wearing a garland of native *maile* around his neck. In one hand he clutches a black leather-bound bible and in the other branches of some tropical botany and a small wooden bowl.

'Friends, brothers, sisters, welcome. We meet here today

for the blessing of ambulance Pawaa 1. We all know why we are doing this, why this rig needs our blessing.'

Except for the visitor, I think to myself, before leaning in toward Tippy and whispering, 'A blessing?'

Tippy nods. 'Actually,' he whispers back, 'more like exorcism.'

Exorcism?

As a paramedic I've been in some pretty bizarre situations, but an ambulance exorcism? It would certainly be my first. No wonder they referred to it as a ritual.

'Haunted?' I whisper again.

'So they say,' he replies.

Many ambulance stations around the world are known to have ghosts, but never had I heard of an ambulance itself possessed by a lingering soul.

'Everybody please hold out your hands,' continues the priest, lifting the little wooden bowl above his head. 'This water fell from the sky twenty-five years ago. It is sacred water of the islands. First, with this water I will wash your hands, wash the healing hands of all EMTs and paramedics, as a symbol of cleansing you from dark thoughts and dark forces surrounding you.'

Every paramedic submits to the blessing. Mitch, Tippy, the others, all of them holding out their hands, the priest anointing each upturned palm with water. When he finishes this, he raises the three long strands of Hawaiian *ti* leaf into the air before dipping them into the holy water and flicking it over the ambulance.

'With these three leaves of *ti,* representing the past, present and future, or the Father, Son and Holy Ghost, whatever your interpretation, Ke Akua we ask your goodness to flood into Pawaa 1, to fill it with your Aloha spirit.'

The priest opens the driver's door of the ambulance, wets his fingers and draws a cross over the Ford logo in the steering wheel.

'Lord Ke Akua, we ask that you bless this steering wheel.'

And then he goes around to the bonnet and slaps it three times with the *ti* leaves and holy water and says, 'Third time's a charm, Ke Akua, bless this rig and chase out evil with your Aloha spirit, Lord.'

The priest circles the ambulance three times, whacking the sides with his leaves and water, slapping the tires and praying that they will 'hold tight to the Aina' – the road. He then takes his bible in both hands and climbs into the back. Muffled, we can near him continue his exorcism.

'Oh, Ke Akua, with this bible written in Hawaiian language, may your word put evil to flight, Lord. Mahalo Ke Akua, Mahalo Ke Akua. Mahalo Ke Akua.'

And with that the blessing is over. It's a relief there has been no sudden rushing wind, flying objects or thrashing about of some hapless human vessel.

'Well?' asks Tippy.

'Great,' I reply, 'Pretty tame for an exorcism, don't you think?'

'As a Christian I'm not really superstitious,' Tippy tells me, 'but there was something seriously present in the back of that ambulance.'

Mitch comes over and says, 'Best thing about a blessing is getting out of the city. We're all meeting at headquarters for a drink, by the way. Tippy, the Chief wants you to drive Pawaa 1 up.'

Tippy freezes to the spot.

'No way am I driving that thing!'

Mitch and I laugh.

'Don't worry,' says Mitch. 'The ghost is gone.'

THE CROSS OF FIRE

Mexico

In the front seat of our ambulance the Christmas *piñata* on my lap is a giant star of gold foil, pink and blue ruffled crepe and streamers, room enough inside for a family of three. Some *piñatas* are so enormous they require transport by flatbed truck and jackhammers to break them. This one, I worry, will be ruined well before Mitzi Garcia's fiesta if our driver Arturo goes on the way he is, hitting a hundred clicks an hour on the Chalma la Villa. One hard brake for a looming speed bump and I fear the cabin will be filled with papier-mâché dust as our fine *piñata* is crushed between my body and the dashboard.

While the siren is loud, even with the windows up, Arturo has the stereo louder still, singing along to Vicente Fernandez, the ultimate mariachi crooner, the Mexican medic's mojo, a living elixir of courage for every ambulance crew. With big band brass he brings them boldly to the scene. With the loneliest of lullabies he serenades the dead.

Our *piñata* blocks my view of the road ahead but out the side I glimpse the Cerro del Chiquihuite mountain and its steep ridge of rough concrete dwellings, closely packed like a Palestinian ghetto, strung together by a tangled web of powerlines hung with hijacked running shoes and shredded plastic bags. A few houses in most streets have city-facing walls painted in primary colours, a Mexican tradition not everyone can afford. But despite the poverty of Tlalnepantla and surrounding colonies, many residents have put up Christmas lights and blinking reindeers, making for a wonderful view at night when even a slum can look pretty in the sparkling dark. Castillo Chico, San Juanico and San Antonio are all places served by the Lazaro Cardenas Red Cross, colonies of low income, unemployment and regular violence. While no part of Mexico City compares with the narco bloodshed of the northern towns, *paramédicos* at the Red Cross Delegation of Lazaro Cardenas see their fair share of gunshots and stabbings and other types of penetrating trauma known as *perforados* – the perforated.

Arturo speeds along Puerto Mazatlan, pushing the Ford Econoline to its limit. As the V8 roars off every speed hump, memories of my own days driving an F100 ambulance in outback Australia flood back. The gutsy sound of the engine, that surge of a mighty power and the thrilling scent of petrol I didn't have to pay for. Arturo is a man pining for speed, infuriated by the menace of Mexico City's countless speed humps, as frequent as every thirty metres on some roads and each a foot high. These necessitate bringing the ambulance to a complete standstill and creeping up and over every hump. No wonder the Mexicans say that 'your pizza comes quicker than your ambulance'. Widespread distribution of Domino's outlets and their fleet of delivery bikes may have something to do with this. Most speed humps have a narrow gap in the middle through which motorbikes can easily pass without stopping. While the city's speed-breakers have probably prevented numerous fatalities, they also double the time it takes for ambulances to reach accidents. Responses are rarely quicker than twenty minutes, often more than thirty, and cause me to speculate that these humps may well have led to just as many deaths as they were built to prevent.

On the Vista Hermosa a young boy leaving school has been the victim of a vicious act of bullying and thrown into the path of a delivery truck by his classmates. We pull up through a few hundred onlookers. It's another feature of Mexican accident scenes, that are, for most people, a spot of free entertainment.

Luckily the lad has come out of his ordeal with no more than a couple of limb fractures, leaving his head, neck and torso intact. On this same road a week earlier, a middle-aged man was rolled into a ball of flesh and denim as the jeep he was struck by kept on driving for another kilometre or so. It's a good thing the boy isn't critical as our time on scene is considerably delayed while we wait for the owner of the truck to arrive. Compulsory third party insurance does not exist in Mexico and according to the law, if the owner of the vehicle involved is not insured and does not agree to pay for the ambulance ride and hospital costs of the casualty, the driver of the vehicle will be sent to jail. And in this case, it happens. The owner of the truck turns up and shrugs. He has no interest in paying for the boy's treatment. Police then inform the poor truck driver he will be locked up, indefinitely, even though none of it was his fault. In a city where ten thousand drivers are looking for work, it's cheaper for the owner to let his driver rot away behind bars and simply hire another one. Meanwhile, the patient and his mother – who has by now arrived on the scene – are informed that no one will be covering their medical expenses. Rarely have I seen such a miserable and angry bunch of people at one relatively minor pedestrian accident. Only in rural India and Pakistan, where drivers who hit pedestrians can be lynched on the spot by angry village mobs, could an outcome be worse for a driver than years in a Mexican prison.

My long-time friend Mitzi Garcia Rodriguez, a *paramédico* with the Red Cross for more than ten years, is twenty-six years old and has incredible ambition for a single mother of a baby girl. She works for the government as a disaster response officer while simultaneously completing a degree in forensic criminology, En Ciencias Juridicas y Criminologicas. Any time she has left is devoted to volunteering on the ambulances of Lazaro Cardenas, where she does just about as many hours as a full-time paramedic in other parts of the world. She's a beautiful woman and taller than the average Mexican; her most striking feature being her unusual hazel-green eyes, accentuated with smoke-grey eye shadow. At every few sets of traffic lights she touches up her lips with a cherry-red lipstick. It's no coincidence that whenever Mitzi is on shift she's always offered the front seat of the ambulance, and at most hospitals a bed for her patients in less than ten minutes, even when the wards are overflowing. For these reasons, along with her playful, optimistic personality, she is the ideal paramedic partner to have in Mexico City.

Christmas Eve is a day away and the *colonias* are bustling with crowds shopping in the local markets for decorations and presents, kegs of apple cider and tequila, sweets enough to fill their enormous *piñatas* and food for the midnight feast. It's hard not to notice the poverty as we crawl through the markets by ambulance. And yet those living on these outskirts of Ciudad de Mexico are ready to party as hard, if not harder, than every other Mexican. From the ambulance I see them, the residents of Lazaro Cardenas, preparing their steep mountainside streets for neighbourhood fiestas, stringing tinsel from house to house, watched by scruffy children lounging on the rusty wrecks of Volkswagen Beetles, fishing sliced melon from little plastic bags.

Some teenage girls in velvet tracksuits and tightly plaited hair – probably *reggaetoneros*, those kids obsessed with reggaeton music – are plucking chilli peppers from a roadside tree and eating them like grapes. Brightly painted shrines to various Catholic saints, some six-feet tall and smothered in garlands of tinsel, their holy faces powdered with silvery glitter flashing in angled rays of afternoon sun, are encased behind glass and get particular attention this time of year. In addition to these suburban shrines collectively maintained, most families, even the poorest, will install an elaborate nativity diorama in their private homes. Some of them devote an entire room to three-foot Mary and Joseph statues, shepherds and lambs, wise men and guiding stars, all doing their thing on blankets of Astroturf or hay.

Arturo takes us into the backstreets of Zona Escolar, past houses with lazy old musicians playing guitars out front, children flicking marbles and waving at the ambulance as we pass. Before long we pull up at the end of a cul-de-sac and Mitzi jumps out to pick up her daughter Maria José from kindergarten. Once inside the ambulance, the little girl clambers all over the stretcher still lightly stained with the blood of the last shooting victim. Mitzi pulls out a picture book about frogs and reads it to her on the way home. Seeing Mitzi playing with Maria José makes me momentarily homesick for Kass and Paloma, celebrating Christmas back in Sydney without me. Fifteen minutes later we have dropped Maria José to Mitzi's mother's place where she will stay until Mitzi has finished her shift.

We return to Lazaro Cardenas and drive around a man under a car in the middle of the road, fixing it right there and then where it has broken down. This scene reminds Arturo that the brake pads on our ambulance need changing before the mechanics disappear for Christmas. It's an important matter as almost the entire catchment belonging to Lazaro Cardenas is built along a very steep mountainside. Some streets are so precipitous that no vehicle is able to ascend them at all. Both Mitzi and Arturo have dealt with many horrific trauma cases directly caused by the failing of brakes on these inclines. Indeed, only last week a tanker on the other side of the mountain toppled over and slid down a slope, demolishing everything in its path, killing thirteen people. Most cities of the world would consider such an event to be cause for national mourning. In Mexico City, however, a major incident occurs every other day. Understandably, the last thing Arturo wants is for the brakes on our ambulance to fail and create an equal horror. Judging by the way he drives there's every possibility. Not a case goes by that isn't accompanied by the smell of smoking rubber and, later, the sounds of squeaking and crunching and locking up. Arturo may insist to me the brake pads on the ambulance are replaced once a month, but I've seen the fitting of new pads twice in a single week. And now again, third time in a fortnight. Crazy! None of us minds, of course. So long as the ambulance is up on the hoist, we're off-line and kicking back and hearing the story again about the man who got his lower leg traumatically amputated by a train last month and complained about a painful foot. 'Don't lie to me,' Arturo apparently told him. 'You don't *have* a foot.'

When the ambulance is done we head off to a dying woman in a blue room of crucifixes. There are twenty or thirty relatives conducting a bedside vigil. They all just sit and stare hypnotically at each breath, watching and waiting, every now and then getting up to turn the page of an open Bible on which her head has been rested. An amber rosary is wound around her fragile fingers, as if preventing an escape from her impending demise.

As we leave the house, one of the daughters tries slipping us a few hundred pesos. Instinctively I shake my head but Mitzi takes it and thanks her. Back at the ambulance I challenge Mitzi on the ethics of accepting the money. Taking cash from a loaded Kuwaiti is one thing, but a poor Mexican?

She shrugs. 'We cannot *ask* for it but if they want to *give* it to us, we are permitted to take it.' This makes me laugh. Artful lingering is by no means the reserve of hotel porters, as I learnt on the job in London.

En route back to the station we stop off to buy chicken tacos, black coffee and cigarettes from our little donation. It's not much but it will help us through the night ahead. We've already been at work for twelve hours and have another thirty-six to go. Yes, it's a truly painful thought for a paramedic used to complaining about fatigue a minute or so after the twelfth hour. Mexican shifts of forty-eight hours straight are completely new to me and may, for some remote village ambulance service, be a fine idea. But in a city of twenty million served by less than thirty emergency ambulances, it equals a total lack of sleep for two whole days and nights. By the fortieth hour, ambulances in Mexico City are weaving all over the road, the paramedics inside them trying their best to make the muttering of gibberish sound like clinical advice. If fatigue has reached a critical point, some *paramédicos* have been known to abandon the sorry charade of functionality altogether and climb onto the stretcher to grab some sleep beside their patients.

Come to think of it, no wonder Arturo sounds drunk even when he isn't.

The ambulance station at Lazaro Cardenas on Calle Alpino is a two-storey building, as run-down as the rest of the neighbourhood and flanked by a small 24-hour Red Cross clinic staffed by a doctor and a pair of registered nurses in paper bonnets. Our occasional periods of downtime are often spent hanging out here with these nurses, sipping hot Christmas punch full of guava and sugarcane that simmers away in a big pot on a corner stove. The clinic's doctor, Dagoberto Rodriguez – better known as Dr Baloo because of his jolly bear-like build – joins ambulance crews on

Saturdays and Sundays after a week in the clinic. It's an excessive commitment and difficult to understand given that he's limited in the medications he can use while working on ambulances. Unfortunately, the norms laid down by the Health Secretariat of Mexico are vague and imprecise when it comes to medications permitted for use in the pre-hospital setting. Paramedics administer little more than IV fluids and glucose drips and even these they do without official backing from the Red Cross. All Dr Baloo ever dares carry with him are a few ampoules of adrenalin 1:10,000 and vials of Atropine slipped into the top pocket of his uniform shirt should he ever come across a cardiac arrest. This, he knows, is most unlikely as cardiac arrests are rarely encountered by Mexican ambulance crews. Mitzi Garcia, for instance, has only performed CPR four times in ten years and on these occasions it was done at gunpoint. Literally. Nor is she the only Mexican paramedic to have been forced into a hopeless resuscitation by criminal gang members who fail to grasp that a man riddled with fifty bullets, decapitated or sawn in half is usually well beyond revival.

Ambulances are never called to patients with chest pain but rather when the heart of the patient with chest pain finally gives out. If someone collapses without a pulse, the Mexico City ambulance response times of greater than twenty minutes precludes the initiation of resuscitation due to the near-zero possibility of a save. None of the Red Cross ambulances are equipped with a defibrillator anyway. Poor public education, slack response times and no defibrillators means that Mexico at any time of day is far worse a place to suffer a heart attack than Venice during high tide.

'People only call for two things in this city,' says Dr Baloo, slurping on his punch. 'When someone can't be woken and when they see lots of blood. In both cases there's a good chance the patient will be dead by the time we get there.'

How jealous those young, super keen paramedics back home

would be as they respond around the clock to teenagers feeling depressed, men with toothaches and women with period pain. In Mexico, when a call comes in, it's probably 'the big one'.

At Ticoman, near the Cinemax, a man has fallen – or been thrown – from the seventh floor of a building into a central atrium, landing in a garden, tangled in a washing line, bleeding onto clothes that were hung out to dry. An old lady living on the ground floor is so mad at seeing her washing ruined she refuses to allow us in to attend the patient, loudly bolting the door.

'Let him bleed to death!' she yells from the other side.

We have little choice but to summon the rescue squad Escuadrón de Rescate y Urgencias Médicas, known as ERUM, which belongs to the Mexico City Police. ERUM also operates a dozen ambulances in the city, staffed by general practitioners and police drivers, crews that have a reputation for being rather hapless under pressure. Many Red Cross medics view ERUM cynically because it can only attend a small fraction of the emergencies in the city. What ERUM is very good at, however, is search and rescue, and when they arrive the rescuers decide that instead of forcing entry to the old lady's apartment they will use an A-frame and abseil from a window on the second floor.

As the rescue is carried out and we prepare our equipment to remove the patient, an unmarked car with flashing strobes and blinking beacons pulls up outside. From the stairwell window I see a man wearing a paramedic jacket rush in to join the drama. The Star of Life logos on his sleeves are somewhat ambiguous and the stethoscope around his neck is of the budget variety. It is also the only item of medical gear the chap is taking in. What he does carry instead is a collection of expensive digital cameras. While I find this odd, neither Mitzi nor Arturo pay him the least bit of attention. For the duration of the rescue, as the unconscious patient is hoisted up in a Sked stretcher, the man leans out an adjacent window and begins snapping shots of the sorry victim swinging to and fro like a pendulum, bumping into the brickwork.

'He's not Cruz Roja?' I ask Mitzi.

'No,' she says.

'Then who?' I ask.

'A journalist,' she says, matter-of-factly.

'Journalist? Dressed like a paramedic?'

'Sure. It's normal here. They have radio scanners and make their cars like emergency vehicles. This way they find the action.'

Arturo then tells us about a proper ambulance wagon with stretcher and all, staffed by two fake paramedics – a writer and a photographer – operating for a couple of years out of San Juanico. They got the best stories in town, at least the ones involving death and destruction.

Didn't it bother Arturo and his colleagues?

Not at all, he says.

The Red Cross crews knew it was a dangerous game the journalists were engaging in and expected it would ultimately backfire. On the day it did, the fake paramedics happened to arrive first on the scene of a nasty gun massacre and instead of helping out began snapping pictures and scribbling in notepads while victims bled to death on the pavement. Surely it wasn't a surprise when they found themselves promptly set upon by a mob of angry bystanders, necessitating a rescue by genuine Red Cross paramedics. After that no one ever saw the fake ambulance again.

In Mexico, the dead sell the papers. Newsstands across the country are daily galleries of gore, the front pages of twenty-five-cent print editions plastered with montages of gruesome bodies juxtaposed with the occasional naked woman posing in a Santa hat for Christmas. Millions of copies are sold each morning. While I'm ideologically opposed to those who exploit death like this,

I find myself unable to resist peering at the terrible, uncensored images as I pass them on my way to work. There are mutilated victims of crime, faces knifed through the eyes, headless cadavers dumped by state highways. With the narco war offering up a daily body count to rival Afghanistan, there is no shortage of material. Recently, when an oil explosion claimed twenty-eight lives in Puebla, the picture of a charred toddler with a little arm around her blackened mother sent me teary-eyed into metro Tacubaya. It seems no horror is too despicable for publication in the Mexican papers. But although it disturbs me, I'm fascinated all the same by my own reaction, compelled by my irresistible morbid curiosity, one I share with every other human, even those who act so indignantly about this type of trashy photojournalism.

As a lover of photography I have for many years been a fan of Enrique Metinides, the Mexican news photographer and the artistic, haunting images of tragedy he has compiled over five decades following paramedics in Mexico City. Many of these are now major collectors' items, regularly exhibited in prestigious galleries of Paris, London and New York. His photos convey the most extreme and dramatic moments of crisis or horror in a single and often beautifully atmospheric frame.

Notwithstanding his artistic talents, Metinides is, without a doubt, the key figure in defining the Mexican genre of journalism known as *nota roja*, the school of sensationalists. Like the fake paramedic who turned up to our trauma case, Metinides also monitored a Red Cross radio day and night. He knew many ambulance workers by name and is said to have in his apartment on Avenida Revolucion one of the largest collections of model ambulances in the world. If I respect Metinides as an artist, how can I criticise the latter-day *nota roja* who make their living chasing ambulances? They are, after all, giving the people what they want. As a paramedic I am in some ways fortunate to have a regular means of satiating any morbid curiosity existing within me.

Although I may glance in passing at the front pages of *El Graffico*, *El Metro*, *Alarme* and other Mexican newspapers plastered with gore, I have no desire at all to buy and peruse them, just as I don't watch horror films. But if the multitudes of bystanders who gather around every accident I attend as a paramedic are anything to go by, it's clear that human beings are fascinated by catastrophes that befall others. The accident or violent crime could, after all, have happened to them.

'A manager at the Red Cross used to own one of those papers,' Mitzi mentions as we cruise back to the station. 'His staff were told to get as many pictures of bodies as possible.'

Seeing the expression on my face, Mitzi shrugs in her non-plussed way. 'You're surprised?' she asks.

I suppose not. In Mexico, corruption, nepotism and conflict of interest are widespread and entrenched within every sector of the government and business. Why would the Red Cross be any different? Where is all the money from Geneva and local donations ending up? Why is it the paramedics of the Cruz Roja have to repair their own ambulances, buy their own uniforms, supply their own equipment, work without oxygen or drugs or proper neck collars, and ration their use of examination gloves to three pairs a shift? Don't use your gloves too early, they often remind me. It's the golden rule. You'll regret it if you get a gunshot at three in the morning. Who in the world wants to work on ambulances in this bloodbath of a country without gloves, all for a monthly paycheck of US$300?

'You can't blame us for trying to make a bit of money on the side,' says Mitzi. 'There are many ways a paramedic can do it here at the Red Cross, I've told you.'

The tips don't cut it most days. Indeed, there are better means to earn a little extra. Funeral parlours are one. If we get a deceased – and this is sometimes every second case – a quick call to the local funeral director can attract a handsome commission. Failing that, photos of the bodies, even those taken with a mobile phone, can earn 200 pesos from any number of newspapers. A nasty corpse with a weapon embedded in it, for example, or creatively mutilated or crawling with maggots, may even get the front page. This is worth about 500 pesos, approximately US$50, cash in hand.

'Paramedics who do this, we call them *morboso*,' says Mitzi, although I suspect she qualifies as a *morboso* herself given the galleries of dead bodies on her Facebook page.

'At least,' she goes on, 'these paramedics don't steal from patients.'

Well, yes, that is a good thing. Mitzi makes this point because she knows that all I hear around town is that Mexican paramedics are petty thieves who will pinch the wallet of an unconscious patient or slip the family jewellery into their underpants. I've never witnessed this and the medics at Lazaro Cardenas strongly deny they have ever engaged in such criminal activities, tempting as it may be for those trying to feed their families on insubstantial paypackets.

'We might be *loco*,' says Arturo, 'but some things, like stealing from patients, we will never do.'

He goes on to tell me that paramedics belonging to some other, private ambulance services are apparently the ones known to rob casualties and muddy the reputation of the rest. With almost no regulation of EMS in Mexico, it is not inconceivable that several of the dozen private ambulance companies operating around the city may have been set up for the sole purpose of gaining unparalleled access to people's homes and back pockets.

At the church of San Pedro Xalostoc, reached by pushing through a busy market selling fruit and vegetables and little baby Jesus dolls, we are shown to a woman in her forties, collapsed unconscious with very shallow respirations. She lies barefoot and dishevelled under the impassive gaze of a six-foot Mary.

Dr Baloo, whom we picked up from the station on our way past, gives her a vigorous shake, but nothing happens.

'PVC,' he mutters, suspecting the patient has sniffed too much PVC glue, one of many inhalants commonly abused by those too poor to afford the amphetamines that travel through Mexico on their way to the United States.

I decide to show Dr Baloo my special pinch, the one I do behind a patient's arm. It wakes the dead, I tell him. But I do it as hard as I can and the woman doesn't flinch.

Mitzi crouches beside me and I sense she is amused.

'Let *us* teach *you* something,' she whispers.

With that she puts down her first-aid kit and opens it. Out of it she takes a bottle of 96 per cent alcohol and calmly pours some onto a ball of cotton wool, allowing it to soak through completely. Then she leans over, pulls open the patient's right eye and squeezes it in.

Just like that, a cruelty of the highest order.

I'm stunned once again. This agonising technique to wake the unconscious makes the ammonia sticks of American paramedics or the face-slapping of Venetian doctors look like true love.

But it doesn't end there.

Unsatisfied with the one feeble grunt of pain from our victim, Mitzi tips some more of the near-pure alcohol into a nasal delivery pump, rams it up the patient's nose and squirts twice, no, three times, until a cry of agony escapes the woman's open mouth like the howl of an injured dog, quickly drowned by spluttering and choking sounds as the alcohol hits her throat.

It's getting dark and back at the station a friendly, well-groomed medic Juan-Carlos Barrera, along with Guadalupe, our buxom controller, goad our crew into a *hacer bolita*, known in English as a 'stacks-on', whereby everyone throws themselves on top of one another until we're all lying in a heap of bodies on the tiled floor, or, as Mitzi puts it, a mountain of people. This is fun about once, and only if you're not at the bottom of the pile. It's a curiously juvenile game and much to my dismay there's a 'stacks-on' just about every time we get back to station.

In no way does the fun stop there though. Once we've brushed ourselves down, Guadalupe leads us into a round of *la lupita* in which a paramedic is randomly – sometimes intentionally – singled out and everyone else assembles to strike them as hard as they can on the bottom with a long leg splint. *La lupita* may not be in the league of Scrabble or chess for expansion of the mind, but the staff of Lazaro Cardenas seem to enjoy every moment. While I'm relieved they're all too polite to spank their guests, it's awkward when I find the splint in my own hands and poor Guadalupe bending over in front of me, expecting a whack.

When I do it, I do it gently of course, almost a dummy-smack, which makes everyone cheer and Guadalupe giggle in delight.

Muy loco, I think to myself.

'Before you leave,' mumbles Arturo, lighting a Marlboro, 'we hope you will reach the status of Mexican paramedic.'

This I find rather funny to hear, particularly following a session of their crazy antics, because I'm still unsure how Mexican paramedics can actually earn their 'status' with less than a year's training part-time.

'We're watching you,' he goes on, all of a sudden uncharacter-istically earnest, tapping a filthy aquarium containing the station's goldfish, looping lazily round a sunken galleon with a Red Cross on its sail. 'We're watching and deciding.'

'Deciding? Deciding what?'

Arturo says something in Spanish to the others who all seem taken aback to hear it. In no time at all, an incomprehensible argument has ignited around me. Mitzi has never looked so serious and wags her finger at Arturo while Guadalupe shakes her head and yells and looks at me with pity. It's moments like this I wish I'd stuck with my community college Spanish lessons.

When it dies down, Mitzi turns and says, 'Arturo is making a suggestion. If we think you are good enough to be Mexican paramedic, we will give you the ceremony.'

'The ceremony?'

'Actually, I think in English you call it different.'

'Yes?'

'Yes. I think in English you call it *initiation*.'

'You have an initiation?'

'Of course.'

'To be a Mexican paramedic?'

'Yes. It's called *Cruz de Fuego*. It's meaning is the Cross of Fire. It is a great honour. Only paramedics who graduate from the course and prove themselves in the *colonias* will get the *Cruz de Fuego*. Not everyone is getting the *Cruz de Fuego*. Understand?'

'And what happens when you get it?' I ask her.

'You lie down on the stretcher. We take 96 per cent alcohol and paint big cross on your chest with it, from here to here,' she says, passing her hand from her jugular notch almost to her belly button, crossed by a line from one axilla to the other. 'Then, we light it, and we let it burn, the burning cross, *Cruz de Fuego*.'

No one says anything. They're all staring at me, gauging a reaction, not sure how I'll take the notion of this severe rite of passage.

'It must hurt,' I say.

Mitzi nods. 'Depending on how long we leave it to burn. We all stand round to slap out the fire. If we like you we will do it quickly. And, if we don't like you, maybe we let it burn longer, maybe until you are screaming.'

I ask her if she has received the Cross of Fire herself, and she nods. Suddenly the idea of whacking a female colleague with a splint is child's play.

'Any scars?'

'Sometimes. One paramedic from Polanco, he had a giant red cross on his chest for a year. He also had other problems because his hair and ears caught fire. But we are more careful at this delegation.'

When my spinning mind comes back to earth I find both my hands are instinctively covering my chest. It has, until now, been my ultimate desire that paramedics belonging to every service in which I work will accept me as one of their own. In saying that, I never expected to meet a bunch of medics who would only properly acknowledge me as a brother if I let them set me on fire.

Not wanting to be impolite, I say, 'I'll think about it.'

Arturo laughs. 'No, no! *We* will think about it!'

'So, I don't have a choice?'

'If we decide you get it,' says Mitzi, 'then you get it. If we decide you don't get it, then you can walk away. But if you walk away, you are not a paramedic.'

At least not by Mexican standards, I'm tempted to add.

Juan-Carlos answers a call and Mitzi Garcia looks over his shoulder to see what he is scribbling on a notepad.

'*No está mal,*' says Mitzi, 'Nothing too serious, just a woman hit by a car on one of the highways.'

At first I interpret her flippancy as typical paramedic humour. Then, as I sit for the next few minutes on my own in the dark front seat of the ambulance and wait for some indication that we are, in fact, responding to the woman hit by a car, I begin to wonder if Mitzi was telling the truth. I wait and wait for our departure, imagining our poor patient sprawled on lane five, embedded in the bitumen. Behind the lace curtains I see one of the medics lighting a new cigarette while another stares blankly at a Mexican soap on television. Guadalupe is sitting at the coffee table with a pair of scissors, fashioning neck collars from old cardboard boxes. Last I heard, Mitzi had gone to the toilet for a 'quick one'. And as for Arturo, who prefers driving, he's always the last one to leave. He belongs to that school of 'making up time on the road', whereby the longer it takes to get out the door the faster one is permitted to drive while heading to the case. Indeed, whenever the Red Cross crew finally piles into the Ford and heads off, we reach frightening speeds.

Despite this, and even if the paramedics slid down a fire pole like they do in Iceland, our response times would still be atrocious considering the distances and traffic conditions of this chaotic metropolis. Thank goodness there's no reputation to uphold, no widely promoted Pakistani pledge to reach the scene in seven minutes. It helps too that no ambulance service or governing body collects data or sets a response-time standard. And only Domino's pizza have a money-back guarantee if they fail to reach a caller in half an hour, leading some people to conclude that a hot pizza in this country is more valuable than a human life.

Knowing just how long it takes to get an ambulance, many locals around Lazaro Cardenas decide to drive their sick or injured to the ambulance station itself, dropping them on the doorstep. This happened a few nights ago when the explosions of pre-Christmas firecrackers going off were indistinguishable from the sound of pistol shots. Just as I put my head down on a filthy pillow for a wink of sleep there came a screeching of tyres outside and the *clomp* of a body hitting the concrete. He was still alive too, a heavily tattooed young man with several stab wounds to the chest and neck, lucid enough to tell us he'd been axed with an icepick. Who in a city overflowing with dirt-cheap small arms would opt for an icepick? Moreover, as temperatures rarely reach zero here, who would even have an icepick handy?

We leave Arturo behind, sleeping in one of the bunks. Juan-Carlos, Mitzi and I pull up on Federal Highway 85 where a middle-aged woman is lying on the roadside surrounded by a throng of bystanders. Traffic is so fast along this stretch none of us imagines our patient to be suitable for anything but a body bag. We're wrong. The old lady is confused but conscious, face glistening with tears in our flashing red and blues.

As paramedics we ought to avoid making patients feel stupid about their poor judgment. On the other hand, we like going home with answers. That's why Mitzi cannot resist asking our patient what possessed her to cross an eight-lane highway at night swathed in a black woollen shawl. But her reply is to ask us where she is, which she does every minute or so after that for the rest of our time together.

Juan-Carlos brings the only neck collar from the ambulance – a plastic and foam thing used a good three hundred times before, scuffed and stained and bent out of shape. Nothing's disposable at the Mexican Red Cross, I remember.

Mitzi looks up. 'What about the cardboard ones?'

'We forgot to get some off Guadalupe,' replies Juan-Carlos.

'Then we won't use anything at all,' she says, a little annoyed.

Her rationale makes sense. I've seen this particular collar before. When applied, it puts the head way off the midline, kinking the neck. Better no collar than a crooked one.

Our patient appears to have every long bone in her body fractured. Her pelvis is most probably split in two, she has shortening-and-rotation to the right leg, bilateral compound tibias, possible fractures of both upper and lower arms, pain over the right chest on inspiration, a tender abdomen with sharp increase of pain in the upper left quadrant, cervical and thoracic back discomfort and several deep lacerations and skin tears. In spite of all this, her respiratory rate, pulse and blood pressure are within normal boundaries and she remains conscious during our primary examination. In pre-hospital care, however, complacency is the medic's undoing. I'm under no illusion about that. Our patient's condition is extremely tenuous, especially given her age and mechanism of her injuries. In most ambulance services worldwide she'd be classified as a trauma case of a high priority, but in Mexico City a conscious patient with acceptable vital signs is just not considered critical enough, even if every bone in their body is broken.

Once splinted and loaded up, we sit in the ambulance for an age while Juan-Carlos waits for the Polanco control room to find a hospital willing to accept our patient.

Mitzi cannulates the woman and slowly drips in Hartmann's solution. It's all she's got to give, if one doesn't count reassurance. 'Without pain relief we become very good at that,' she once told me. I've seen her work marvels on screaming patients using gentle words alone. Meanwhile, in systems where analgesia is a whimper away, paramedics can avoid any more than a brief exchange with their patients before knocking them out with an opiate.

Playing on faith is also a common strategy in Mexico, as it is in Italy, where ambulance nurses cannot autonomously give analgesia. And how bizarre it is to hear a faithless paramedic reminding a patient about the suffering of Christ, using striking imagery of a beaten Jesus dragging his crucifix to Golgotha. And yet these visualisations are surprisingly effective in relieving patients' pain, even the most severe.

That said, the inability of Mexican paramedics to administer medications is something they compare to firemen being asked to work without water. Their training course may be just a year, but a year is time enough to learn about what can save a life. A year is enough to learn that a man with a heart attack can be saved by aspirin, that a child suffering anaphylaxis will survive with adrenalin, that a patient having an asthma attack may pull through with nebulised Salbutamol.

There are many theories among Cruz Roja staff as to why they are unable to administer anything. Most common is the reference made to the Mexican appetite for drugs – and they don't mean cocaine. One only has to turn on the television to see almost every advertisement features pills or sprays or therapeutic solutions for every imaginable and imagined complaint. Neon-lit *farmacias*, grand as casinos, loom over intersections all around the city, open twenty-four hours and forever brimming with people in pyjamas and dressing-gowns. They are like enormous candy shops for adults; only the United States self-medicates more vigorously than Mexico. My colleagues are the first to admit that drugs issued to paramedics wouldn't last a week. There'd be a party in the ambulance on a Friday night and by sunrise all would be gone. As for medications with undesired recreational effects, these would be re-sold on the black market to supplement dismal wages.

Expanding the pharmacological reach of paramedics under the supervision of a medical director is hard, too, when most Red Cross paramedics are volunteers. Providing an essential service for a city of twenty million is a massive task requiring enormous numbers of volunteers, day and night, all year round. Sometimes when an ambulance service is this desperate for staff, it may take on individuals who do not possess the highest clinical ability. Services failing to remunerate top-quality professionals adequately will always have difficulty attracting and retaining them. After all, not every qualified paramedic is motivated by a deep-seated benevolence. To plenty of ambulance workers it's a job like any other, allowing them to provide for their families and build a future. And while most of my colleagues at Lazaro Cardenas are truly dedicated and intelligent, this cannot be said about every member at every delegation. No doubt the policy-makers of the Mexican Red Cross have asked themselves many times just how safe it would be to provide their staff with potentially lethal drugs.

A service known for its rationing of latex gloves could hardly afford drugs anyway. That the Red Cross is capable of responding to the endless barrage of 065 calls, operating the primary EMS for a place as large as Mexico City, is already impressive. Why should it bankroll multi-million dollar advanced pre-hospital care that in most other cities of the world is funded by the government? Shouldn't responsibility for ambulance service provision rest with the state? While the police-run ERUM has existed for many years, everyone knows it fails to meet public demand. No wonder the government has avoided setting any ambulance regulations or establishing key performance indicators. It couldn't possibly meet them.

Twenty minutes later we are still waiting. Mitzi tells me to jump out and ask Juan-Carlos in the front seat what's going on. I walk around and see him shaking his head, tapping the radio. When he notices me he asks, *'Teléfono? Teléfono?'*

Evidently the ambulance radio has malfunctioned and I hand him my mobile phone. He dials up the control centre for a lengthy and heated argument. Finally, leaving the engine running, he gets out, goes to the back of the ambulance and informs Mitzi we are heading to the Ruben Leñero Hospital at least forty-minutes' drive away in order to be assessed, then, after that, to the Gregorio Salas hospital to have X-rays done, and finally driving on to Balbuena for a possible admission.

Three hospitals? Mitzi rolls her eyes. 'All of them in opposite directions of Mexico City,' she says, cursing.

We speed off up the highway, our patient bumping up and down on the hard spine board over each pothole. She slides from side to side round every bend in the road, yelling out in agony each time, gripping her broken hip with her broken arm, trying to calm herself with Hail Marys.

Suddenly we slow down and out of the sliding window I see the illuminated sign of a petrol station. Juan-Carlos pulls in and cuts the siren. Typical, I think to myself. Not an hour ago, sandwiched between Juan-Carlos and Mitzi in the front seat, I'd pointed out to them how low the petrol gauge was reading, which both of them shrugged off. Now, carrying a patient in unrelieved pain, we stop and fuel up with our emergency lights still flashing. At least, I think to myself, we haven't actually *run out* of petrol altogether, which Arturo did *twice* last week, leaving us on the outskirts of some dangerous colony as he took off with a jerry can and hitched a ride to the nearest service station. Once the five litres of petrol from the jerry can had been added to the tank, we were back on the road. I wondered why Arturo did not immediately fill up after that, but said nothing. Sure enough, half an hour later, we ran out of petrol again, this time on the way to an unconscious male.

Perhaps Juan-Carlos should not have left the beacons on. Perhaps he should have left the engine running back at the scene. I don't know.

But once refuelled he's unable to start the ambulance.

Our battery is flat and we're not going anywhere.

Mitzi sighs and rolls her eyes again.

She takes another blood pressure.

'Push, push!' calls Juan-Carlos, opening the rear doors to let me out. 'Come, *señor*, we need push, push, pushing!'

Try as we might, the service station attendant and I are unable to generate near enough momentum for a clutch start. Everything comes to a halt with a jerk and a sharp squawk from the patient, followed by silence.

'*Teléfono! Teléfono!*' demands Juan-Carlos.

I hand him my phone a second time. He makes a call and lights a cigarette and once more we are waiting.

Fifteen minutes go by until we hear a siren coming down from Ticoman and see the revolving reds of another ambulance rapidly approaching. Seems Arturo, woken from his nap, has driven the other Ford from the station. Without getting out he pulls in behind us. I stay in the front seat and watch in the side mirror as Arturo edges forward until his fender butts up against our rear bumper with a jolt, eliciting another cry of pain from the back of the wagon. Juan-Carlos lets off the handbrake and Arturo pushes us forward with the second ambulance until we get enough speed to start. The engine kicks in and Juan-Carlos revs it hard. Back on goes the siren and we're off again, giving Arturo a wave for his trouble as we speed away.

After half an hour we arrive at the first hospital and wait for our patient to get a doctor's opinion. This takes a while because the doctor is typing up his last patient's notes on a 1940s Remington typewriter, constantly making mistakes, cursing and pulling out the paper and starting over with ever more aggressive tapping.

Once finished there, we transfer our patient to a hospital where X-rays will be taken and onward to Balbuena for offloading. Not one of the hospitals we visit gives her a shot of morphine or any other analgesia and by the time we reach our ultimate destination it is four hours since the woman actually suffered her accident. She now appears pale and disorientated and lethargic. We are most relieved finally to lift her onto a bed in the orthopaedic ward of Balbuena.

After a midnight hamburger and now rolling home, I ask Mitzi if we can stop at a corner store up ahead to buy a drink.

'Are you mad?' she says. 'This is Tepito. We don't get out of the ambulance in Tepito, we don't even slow down in Tepito. People are shot in Tepito for nothing.'

The streets out my window are heaped with garbage, but there is no one about.

'I don't see anyone at all.'

'That's because no one comes here after dark.'

'Well, if no one's here after dark, who's going to shoot me?'

'They're watching, they'll jump out,' says Mitzi.

'Come on!' I protest.

'Try it,' she says, and Arturo slows down.

'Nah, it's okay,' I say. 'I don't need a drink anyway.'

For the rest of the journey home we swap stories about cases we have been to, which is something I shouldn't bother engaging in with paramedics like these. My worst job in fifteen years could never outdo Mitzi's recollection of arriving first at a massacre in which a man had opened fire with his machine-gun, killing twelve people in under a minute.

A savage wrestling match is going on when we arrive at station. We hear the sounds of crashing and whooping while reversing the ambulance in. Much like the masked *luchadores* who fight every Friday night at Arena Mexico, there are few rules at Lazaro Cardenas and plenty of broken furniture whenever the paramedics have a grapple. As Mitzi opens the door Guadalupe is launching from a stool. For a moment she seems suspended in mid flight, her head turning to look at us before she lands stomach down on top of poor Arturo spreadeagled on the tiles. Seeing the opportunity, neither Mitzi nor Juan-Carlos hesitate to join in. Immediately they throw themselves on the *hacer bolita*.

Extracting himself from the bottom of the pile, Arturo announces he and Guadalupe are off to do some administration. I'm not sure I've heard them right and turn to Mitzi for clarification. Yes, indeed, she confirms, they are off to do some administration. Anywhere else on the planet at this time, paramedics would be either on a case or tucked into bed. Neither wrestling nor administration occurs after pumpkin hour, unless, it appears, one is working for the Cruz Roja. I tell them I'll be turning in for the night and head upstairs.

An hour later I'm shaken awake by Felipe Domínguez, a junior paramedic with a mischievous face. 'Tequila time, *señor*!' he exclaims excitably.

It takes me a moment to remember. Two days earlier, when the lad turned up for a shift, I asked him how his first-aid kit was so heavy given that Mexican paramedics carry no drugs. Even the oxygen supply was out that week. He was hesitant and sheepish and quiet. So I unzipped the kit in front of him and found therein two full bottles of Jose Cuervo tequila.

'It's 100 per cent Blue Agave,' protested Felipe, expecting my concern would be the quality of the spirit he had chosen.

'For the patient?' I asked, only half-jokingly, remembering Mitzi telling me how good tequila was for her Maria José, rubbed on the infant's gums while teething.

'No, *señor*,' he replied with a smile. 'We can't give patient anything, remember.'

Now the same paramedic drags me out to a Red Cross utility he's left running in the drive. On the back of it a group of paramedic students cling to a roll bar and give me a hearty *Buenos noches!* as I climb in the front seat.

We rumble up the hill towards the Lazaro Cardenas *mercados* that during the day is a bustle of pre-Christmas shopping. Now, in the middle of the night, it's completely deserted. Halfway down a slope away from the market we pull up at a vacant lot behind several ambulances acting as windbreaks for eight paramedics huddled round a fire, some slow-dancing together in its flickering light.

When I get closer I notice everyone is there. Arturo sees me and raises a bottle, yelling 'Administration! Administration!' then he stoops and clutches his sides with laughter. An ambulance stereo is cranked full volume, a manic salsa number only those on amphetamines could possibly dance to. This, and the front strobe of another wagon, makes for an atmospheric outdoor fiesta.

'What about management?' I want to know.

'Management? Management is here!' says Arturo, as

Guadalupe giggles by his side. 'Meet Commander Erasmo Arias, in charge of all Tlalnepantla.'

An older gentleman with a neat goatee shakes my hand. He sways somewhat as he does so and I sense Commander Arias has reached the point where he may, at any time, topple over without warning. For this reason I keep his hand in my grip a little longer than usual. The commander appears most touched by this and takes it as pure affection.

'Oh, *señor*,' he slurs. 'Or should I say *compadre* ... yes, *compadre*. You come from so far away, but in this uniform we are *hermanos*, we are brothers, *compadre*.'

I nod, then look over at Arturo, expecting him to mention that I have not, as yet, suffered the Cruz de Fuego, and therefore am not quite the *compadre* the commander thinks I am. We lock eyes for an instant, and I sense he gets what I'm thinking. But he says nothing.

'Now,' continues Commander Arias, 'have you had before the Tequila Tradicional?'

No, I tell him. I prefer to be sober at work. Then I laugh a little, not wanting to pour cold water on the party by sounding spiritless. Still, I inwardly shudder as my *rakija* hangover in Macedonia springs to mind.

'Ah, *señor*!' comes the commander. 'One sip is nothing. And we are not really on duty anyway, are we?'

This I find hard to believe until, almost on cue, we are interrupted by a trauma call three blocks away. Commander Arias orders everyone to hush while he radios that all the medics in the area are otherwise engaged, unable to attend.

And that is that.

'Now,' he says. '*Feliz Navidad*. It's meaning Happy Christmas. You are not Mexican, so I will tell you, this happiness comes best with Tequila Tradicional.'

All eyes are on me, Arturo's especially keen, and I sense this is part of the test, that I'm even now on the path to the Cross of Fire.

The smooth texture and oak tones of Tequila Tradicional make it by far the best tequila I've tasted, and one that is, my Mexican *amigos* agree, impossible to refuse a second glass of. I have three, and that is enough, knowing my poor tolerance. My *compadres* are at least impressed I've had any tequila at all.

Back in the ambulance I sit on the stretcher with Felipe when, while clutching a bottle of Mexcian beer, he says to me, 'You must be seeing us breaking many rules.'

I nod and smile.

'For example, we are travelling in this ambulance now and we are not wearing helmets.'

Surely the man is kidding?

He is drinking a full-strength beer in his uniform, in the back of an ambulance.

'Do you think badly about us for not wearing the helmets?' he asks sincerely.

I'm laughing too hard to answer him.

Climbing back into my bunk before anyone else, I sleep till the next job nearly two hours later. The call comes in at 4 am, male unconscious on the street, and the irony is not lost on me as I step gingerly over the bodies of unconscious medics lying around the station just to get out the door. My bladder needs relieving but the sound of heavy vomiting from the toilet puts me off. Juan-Carlos is sober enough to drive, he assures us, and Mitzi is the only other paramedic in any shape to treat a patient.

It's a lonely intersection high in the colony, a dark crossing lit by one feeble streetlight, where the man dressed from head to toe in black is curled up in the foetal position. Been at a party, speculates a policeman already on the scene. He flicks his torch across the motionless form. Branches of inky blood spread out from the man's head, growing across the concrete towards our feet. Mitzi walks around the other side.

'*Alguien vio algo?* Any witnesses?' she asks, slipping on a glove. Only one glove is necessary to ascertain a pulse.

The policeman shakes his head.

Convenient, Mitzi is probably thinking. Gun crime is so frequent in these parts that police simply cannot keep up. Proper investigations are never a guarantee. In some cases, police have picked up innocents, at times randomly, and put them away for an act they didn't commit in order to close the case. *Presumed Guilty*, a recent documentary by filmmakers Roberto Hernandez and Geoffrey Smith, claims that 92 per cent of convictions are passed without any physical evidence and that hundreds of prisoners in Mexico are serving time for someone else's crime.

'Can you feel a pulse?' Mitzi asks me, just to double-check. A student of forensic science, she knows it's preferable we don't move a body too much, preserving the evidence. As I slip my hand under the collar of the man I notice how neatly trimmed his moustache is. Even in the soft blue light from the nearest corner and the swinging torch beam, it is the most meticulous of moustaches. Pressing my fingers into the soft groove where his carotid artery would normally be throbbing away, I imagine the sunny scene late on the previous day, the man in his backyard peering into a small mirror hung from a hook, snipping at his top lip with a miniature pair of scissors, stooping, checking, snipping – doing this for half an hour or more. How superb he would look for his neighbourhood party, surprisingly superb, unexpectedly superb, yes. He would make the *chicas* turn, make some other men jealous, wishing they too had spent that extra time snipping their moustaches, that little effort that every girl wishes a man would make.

The half a minute it takes to check a pulse on a dead person is a quiet moment of fancy in which I've long indulged my imagination about their lives and, more specifically, the lead-up to their unplanned demise.

I look at Mitzi and say, 'Yeah, he's dead.'

She smiles. 'Good moustache, hey?'

'An inspiration,' I reply.

The next cadaver, illuminated in the ghostly light of dawn, is lying on his back observed by a group of children on bicycles. He's an older man, who may have been knifed on the way home, though he doesn't seem a likely candidate. As is commonly the case in Mexico, the hunt for a victim's family rather than a hunt for the perpetrator begins at the same time an ambulance is called. This often leads to the inconvenience of having any number of relatives – as close as parents and as distant as second-cousins twice-removed – arriving on the scene all wailing and waving and carrying on.

The dead man's wife and teenage boy are, in this case, surprisingly calm, standing in the shade of a nearby tree, holding each other with sombre faces, saying little. Mitzi gets some details from them while the police call their contractors to take the body. The sun rises quickly over the scene and with it comes the inevitable crowd. Soon after that come the vendors of ice-cream and candy, roasted corn and soda. They can smell the dead miles away. We watch as two men assemble a barbecue on the corner and begin to grill some cacti, ten pesos a pop.

On the afternoon of Christmas Eve I catch the metro downtown in search of a present for Mitzi Garcia. Like all other Mexican families, Mitzi's family will be singing at the stroke of midnight, exchanging gifts and then feasting on a banquet of traditional delicacies. It's her birthday, too, the day after Christmas, an excuse for another party, she says. I have already wrapped some Swiss chocolate, Australian wine and a box of plush mice dressed as mariachis for Maria José. As for Mitzi, she has frequently told me she dreams of owning a pulse oximeter. Pegged to the tip of a finger, toe or earlobe, this handy device provides a rapid reading of the blood's oxygen saturation, displayed as a percentage. Ideally, a person will have an oxygen saturation of at least 95 per cent, while a figure below 90 per cent is a concern. It's a useful, non-invasive tool for paramedics already well equipped with diagnostic gear. As active treatment is limited, gadgets like this one are all a Mexican paramedic can wield in order to look busy. Temperatures and blood sugars are likewise done on trauma patients, not because they are relevant assessments necessarily, but because they help a paramedic feel useful and the patient feel attended to. These tools are almost always personally bought by the paramedics.

For twenty minutes I walk down Motolinia, past the rows of shiny wheelchairs lined up on the plaza next to manikins in lab coats holding freshly polished and newly discounted bedpans. Window shopping for medical equipment in Mexico exists only because so many hospitals are without these basic supplies, the patients often forced to bring their own. But doctors, nurses and paramedics – not to mention journalists posing as them – shop here too, and I see them perusing fancy stethoscopes displayed like jewellery on velvet cushions in glass cabinets. Finally I examine a selection of pulse oximeters ranging between 1000 and 2000 pesos each. A nice blue one, small as a matchbox, grabs my attention and I have it gift-wrapped.

On my return metro journey, a blind man inches forward in the aisle of the careering carriage as adeptly balanced as a tightrope walker, singing in a voice parched by years the beautiful 'La Paloma'. As he does, I conjure up a thousand bloodied fingers going into the pulse oximeter I'm carrying, long after I've left the country. Will it save any lives? I'm doubtful. How could it? If it gives a low reading and Mitzi sees the patient needs oxygen, will oxygen be on hand? There is none of it this month and it's peak season. What about next month? The one after that? I feel for my co-workers and understand that employees and volunteers can only do so much in spite of their enormous dedication to saving lives.

Our baby Jesus doll, a diminutive plaster Christ with blushing cheeks, his little hand raised in a blessing, lies staring up from the folds of a blanket in which we swing him back and forth. Mitzi holds the corner across from me, her father a candle in his palm, her mother Leticia playing mandolin nearby, her sister and cousins dancing with Maria José.

> *Rorro Para Celebrar! El Nacimento del Nino Jesus!*
> *Esos tos ojitos, ya los vas cerrando,*
> *Pero estas mirandio*
> *Todos mis delitos*

Together we sing and rock our baby Jesus, passing our corners round. When we're done, we lie Him on a silver tray and surround Him with little white sweets before placing Him in the middle of the nativity scene set out on milk crates.

Now it's time for presents and, much to my embarrassment, I'm given mine first – a bottle of Mezcal. When Mitzi opens hers and finds the pulse oximeter she claps her hands with excitement and kisses me fair and square on the lips.

'*Muchas gracias!*' she says, stringing the oximeter round her neck like a valuable pendant. 'I will wear it every day and night, even in my sleep!'

After dinner, at about 1 am, Mitzi does her make-up, which takes about half an hour, and puts on her uniform. She gives her family a kiss goodbye and her mother tells her to be careful, reminding Mitzi how worried she gets.

'Do you tell her everything?' I ask Mitzi as we go out.

'Mostly. But she's not worried about the actual job,' she replies. 'My mother doesn't like the men I work with. She says they are the most dangerous thing about my work. But I tell her I can handle them.'

When we arrive at Lazaro Cardenas I have my doubts.

Dr Baloo and Guadalupe are dirty dancing on the coffee table, its legs trembling as their bellies rub and jiggle together. Arturo is manning the stereo, cranking *cumbia* to a deafening level. He is naked from the waist up, waving his shirt around his head like a *charro* lasso. Two other male paramedics I don't recognise are unconscious on the tiles, one clutching a half-eaten *torta*. Strewn around the rest of the station is further evidence of a hard party. Even Mitzi looks briefly alarmed.

What has gotten into them? It's not just a Christmas thing. Mitzi has told me more than once that this is the way her friends behave all year round, that working in the realm of crisis and madness causes them to be like this.

'Crazy blood, crazy games,' she tells me. 'Work hard, play hard.'

'Or play hard at work,' I correct her.

Paramedics are constantly reminded of just how quickly, and senselessly, life is extinguished. It is partly this, I believe, compelling us to live wholly and madly, never to hesitate for long, to seize every moment, to try it all. In a sense we live like some people live who've been told their days are numbered. If you only had a month left, what would you do? Spend all your money? Fly around the world? Throw parties every night? The paramedics of Lazaro Cardenas would certainly throw the parties. While every paramedic sees the tenuousness of life and the ruthlessness of death, as Mexicans they see more of it than most. With this in mind, are their crazy excesses not completely understandable?

'There is only one thing to do,' yells Mitzi over the racket we have stumbled on. She goes to the fridge and hands me a cider. 'Join in.'

Not ten minutes after we've arrived, Juan-Carlos luckily hears the phone and the room stops like a freeze frame until the receiver is down. The party continues after that, but Mitzi, Arturo and Juan-Carlos head for the door, and I'm right behind them.

There's a housing complex well alight on Pepe Guizar. We smell the smoke kilometres away through the open window of the ambulance. Someone's baby Jesus candle may have lit up nativity straw, suggests Arturo. The street below is jammed with close to a hundred evacuated residents who apparently descended a smoke-filled stairwell to exit the building. They are milling about coughing in various tempos and keys. Because smoke inhalation – and more specifically the inhalation of toxic fumes – can lead to lung complications hours after exposure, paramedics advise those who have inhaled anything to be observed in a hospital. Of course, patients rarely want to sit in hospital waiting rooms for hours on end. In cases where dozens of people have inhaled the smoke, this would be simply chaotic anyway.

Unperturbed by the numbers, Mitzi has an idea. I see it as a glint in her eyes.

She says something to Arturo in Spanish who, at the top of his voice, bellows out a command. Before long the crowd has transformed into one enormous, snaking queue.

I glance at Mitzi and she winks.

One by one the people file past our ambulance where Mitzi is standing, holding her new Christmas present – the pulse oximeter. This she attaches for a moment onto the pinky finger of each resident, nodding her approval at the display of a good oxygen percentage, then sends them on their way.

'*Mostrar el dedo! Mostrar el dedo!*' calls Arturo loudly and everyone does as he says, holding up their pinky fingers in readiness. A hundred or so people queuing with pinkies raised may be quite a sight, but they do it obediently and are all intensely curious about the tiny magic device the *señorita paramédico* has in her possession. After fifteen minutes it seems as if the queue will never end. That's when we suspect, quite rightly according to the police, that people Mitzi has already tested are rejoining the queue to get another look at the little magic contraption.

As expected, we don't get home. Call after call comes in. Pedestrians hit, stabbings, firecracker injuries, assaults and falls from balconies. It's a London, New York and Sydney New Year's Eve on adrenalin. The ambulance dispatcher is dishing out the calls as rapidly as an air traffic controller at LAX. By 3 am Christmas guests all over the city, crippled by beer and tequila, are getting into their cars for a perilous drive home. It's while we're crossing from one motor accident to another that we're diverted to a shooting on Alpino Avalancha at the biggest street party in Lazaro Cardenas.

Again we pick up Dr Baloo from the station on the way and chase a police car to the scene.

'Keep head down,' puffs Dr Baloo, still breathless, I imagine, from his Mexican belly dance. 'Stay close.'

Arturo pulls up under a rack of disco lights being hurriedly disassembled onto a street that was, until moments ago, a pumping dance floor. He jumps out and lifts the bonnet, slipping the electric cables off the battery as he always does to prevent the ambulance from being stolen.

With their backs to the walls of houses, solemn faces silently watch us walk to a dark huddle, the circle of death, broken by a policeman leading the way, opening up just a crack to let us in.

The inner core of the circle is flickering with the soft honey light of a candle resting at the head of a young man lying on his back, a candle illuminating the way for the onward journey of his departing soul. His eyes are half open and glazed over.

In near-darkness, his blood is jet black, distinguishable only by the reflection of its wetness, like polished obsidian. Everyone has it under foot, great quantities of fresh blood forming a giant puddle in which all of us are sloshing about.

'A head shot killed him, see it?' says Dr Baloo, pointing to a ragged exit wound at the man's temple.

My colleagues are at first uncertain if the half-dozen bullet holes riddling his thorax and abdomen are entry or exit wounds. This surprises me as the ever-increasing gun trafficking from the United States means Mexican paramedics know plenty about firearms. In the cities of the north, paramedics frequently come across ten or twenty gunshot murders a shift, while Lazaro Cardenas paramedics alone see at least three shootings a week in the handful of streets around their station.

Mitzi shakes her head. 'These are definitely exits, but look strange, very small for exit holes.'

A policeman half rolls the body and I see the entry wounds are barely detectable on the other side. Dr Baloo concludes the man was shot from behind at close range in the dense festival crowd, allowing the shooter to disappear quickly among the dark and dancing revellers.

Standing protectively over the man's body is a woman seething with anger – the dead man's sister.

'Mira a este policía!' she cries. 'Mira evidencia!'

In the palm of her hand she shows us a bullet from a .38 calibre handgun. It somehow seems too pretty and small and golden to be as deadly as it was. She's aware, as all Mexicans are, about disappearing evidence and police cover-ups.

'The truth is in my hands, you bastards! You won't be hiding anything tonight!'

Everyone is waiting for a police response. Who will they pick off the street this time? Who will the fall guy be?

A young boy next to me says 'motherfuckers' about the same time the dead man's girlfriend arrives, plunging and scratching through the crowd, falling on her lover in a wild hysteria, smearing his blood like war paint on her face.

Mitzi catches my eye and gives me her 'let's get out of here' look.

We retreat to the ambulance, head back to station and hose off our boots. Arturo and Mitzi argue about how much it costs to have someone killed in San Juanico compared with Lazaro Cardenas then agree, finally, on 500 pesos, about US$50. Only in a country where getting away with murder is so easy could a contract killing come this cheap.

But Mexicans are sick and tired of the violence, says Dr Baloo. More than 10,000 people have been brutally murdered in the narco war this year alone. Unsurprisingly, not a single colleague of mine is willing to take me for a drive through the mountains of Sierra Madre or a drink in the bars of Ciudad Juarez and Chihuahua, northern cities where kidnapping and executions are rife. Things must be really bad in places that adrenalin-junkie paramedics dare not visit. And with the drug trade estimated to represent around 63 per cent of Mexico's economy, the situation is unlikely to change any time soon.

Mitzi's birthday party is in full swing in the garage of her home on Boxing Day when our ambulance, packed with guests, pulls up. A sun-dried man in a frayed sombrero strums a lively *ranchera* outside her front door. Inside, Mitzi's mother has made a pork and corn kernel *pozole* soup, enough for us all. The paramedics tuck in like it's their first meal for days.

After dinner, a band assembles from the guests – five guitars, two mandolins, a trumpet. Six or seven women join them, their voices strong and united as they sing about the old Mexico, the Mexico of their youth, the Mexico of innocence. All of us take a turn dancing with Mitzi. We spin her around and pass her on and she giggles like a child.

Later, after we have savaged a *piñata*, unleashing a violent riot among the guests with the scattering of sweets, Mitzi demonstrates her commitment to the Cruz Roja again and spends the rest of the afternoon and evening on shift. It is, after all, my last day before I fly home, not that we need another reason to celebrate.

'Please don't worry about me,' says Mitzi when Arturo gets her in an arm lock and drags her to the row of ambulances parked outside the station. Juan-Carlos, Felipe, Guadalupe, Dr Baloo, everyone is there for Mitzi's birthday.

'It's tradition,' says Dr Baloo to me, but I still don't know what is going on. 'They do the same to me on my birthday.'

A spine board is taken out of one of the ambulances and I watch, horrified, as Mitzi is put in a neck brace and strapped firmly down, making only the smallest sounds of protest. Her colleagues then lift her upright and lean the stretcher against a wall. A dozen buckets are filled with ice-cold water and one by one each paramedic throws a bucket over Mitzi Garcia, who screams and spits out the water and struggles in vain to escape. According to Arturo, the self-declared mastermind of terror, the usual practice is to dunk helpless birthday victims headfirst into a 44-gallon drum of water, but on this occasion, due to the presence of an international observer, they have toned it down.

The sun descends and the music rises. Mitzi has towelled herself off and seems at least to have gotten warm again. After some tacos are delivered by a man on a bicycle, any housekeeping Guadalupe or the other girls may have done around station has now been undone.

Before long, after a couple of tequila rounds, I find myself thrown in a chair and held down by Juan Carlos and Arturo while Guadalupe gives me a fully clothed lap dance. She grinds upon my left leg and bumps me with her bottom. And while this is not so frightening, I'm near to panic when she smothers my face with her colossal bosom. Cheers and wolf-whistles surround me as the rest of the medics urge Guadalupe on. Yet there's no distress or disgust from her at all. If anything, she genuinely seems to enjoy unbuttoning my uniform shirt and running her fingers through my hair.

Mitzi unveils a chocolate cream birthday cake bought on the way over. Dr Baloo's eyes light up and he licks his lips. But there's nothing as civilised as eating cake with dainty forks off porcelain plates at Lazaro Cardenas, no. Arturo has other plans. Taking a knife, he slices a large chunk of cake topped with whipped cream and slaps it without ceremony onto my naked chest.

Everyone cheers.

'Lamerlo apagado!' he yells to Guadalupe. *'Torta de Australia!'*

And she begins eating the cake off my body to everyone's great amusement. Of course I don't want to ruin the party by objecting to such a lewd act – it's my host's birthday. Besides, to these men and women, licking cake off a co-worker is good innocent fun.

And so is *el caballo*, a game in which I'm lifted, face up, between two paramedics, one grasping my legs and the other my arms, before I'm ridden like a horse by the others who mount me in a callous human rodeo. *El caballo* is enjoyable for just about everyone except the horse, but I know that on my last night in the Red Cross it's the least bad thing that will happen. Although I yearn after all these weeks to be considered a paramedic with the blood of a Mexican – or, as one friend puts it later, a white man with a brown heart – I cannot deny my trepidation about Arturo Modeno's decision and the painful consequences of acceptance.

Midnight is the time of rituals, both holy and unholy alike, an appropriate time for the *Cruz de Fuego* according to Mitzi, but I'm delirious with fatigue. I've barely slept in forty-eight hours. Since I last closed my eyes I've stood over five dead bodies, downed tequila on shift, carried the sick from mountainsides, been at Christmas and birthday parties, thrown water over my host, almost suffocated in the cleavage of another colleague and had chocolate cream cake licked off my chest.

Everyone goes quiet at ten minutes to the witching hour. They stand up and I stand up and Arturo puts both hands on my shoulders and looks me in the eye.

'Amigo, this is the moment we have been waiting for. Because you are like friend to us, we have made decision. You will get our recognition, our tradition.'

My heart begins to pound. The group gathers in close with serious faces, serious faces I have rarely seen them wear. Guadalupe makes the sign of the cross, kisses the fingers she made it with, whispers a Hail Mary. Mitzi reaches out and grabs Arturo's arm, shaking her head.

'*Por favor, Arturo, ten piedad!* Have mercy!'

But he shrugs her off.

'Don't worry,' Mitzi reassures me. 'I promise we won't let it burn for long.'

Felipe goes to the ambulance and wheels a stretcher in. He locks the wheels. It has a red cross printed on the plastic-covered mattress. It looks like a target, like the mark for some sinister sacrifice. Everyone stares with anticipation, thinking the honour will be lost on me, expecting I will turn and run. But I want to have that Mexican blood, feel it course through my big brown heart and live my life as passionately as they live theirs.

I take off my uniform shirt and hand it to Mitzi.

She clutches it tightly, near enough to dab her tears.

When I lie down I'm as helpless as a patient.

Everyone moves in round me.

Looking up, I see Arturo lift the bottle of alcohol and pour it on a handful of cotton. I feel him paint a cold line from my neck to my navel, then across from armpit to armpit. I hold my breath, notice just for a moment a pulse in my temples and squint my eyes, leaving them open just a slit, just enough to see the silver flash of Arturo's cigarette lighter, and the lick of golden flame descending.

GLOSSARY

ATLS:	Advanced Trauma Life Support
Asystole:	State of no cardiac activity, or 'flatline'
BLS:	Basic Life Support
Cannula:	A tube placed in a vein
CPR:	Cardiopulmonary resuscitation
Cricothyroidotomy:	Incision in throat to make an airway
Cubital fossa:	The elbow pit
Cyanosis:	Blue colour of skin due to low oxygen
Defibrillator:	Machine to shock the heart and terminate arrhythmia
ECG:	Electrocardiograph
EMS:	Emergency Medical Service
EMT:	Emergency Medical Technician
Epigastriam:	Upper region of the abdomen
GCS:	Glasgow Coma Scale
Hypovolaemia:	State of decreased blood volume
ICP:	Intensive Care Paramedic
ICU:	Intensive Care Unit
ILS:	Intermediate Life Support
Intubation:	Placement of a plastic tube into the trachea
Paramedic:	Ambulance clinician trained in emergency care
Pre-hospital care:	Modern definition of ambulance work
Pneumothorax:	A collapsed lung
Thoracostomy:	Incision in the chest to relieve air or fluid
Trauma:	Physical injury to the body
Triage:	Determining the medical priority for patients' treatment
Ventricular Fibrillation:	Uncoordinated spasm of heart muscle

ACKNOWLEDGEMENTS

The events, encounters and observations in this book are drawn from my experiences over a period of fifteen years. While all the material presented has been factual, for the sake of narrative coherence, these stories have not always been presented in chronological order, and on numerous occasions I have combined several conversations into one. Likewise, the chapters in this book are not arranged in the actual sequence of my visits to the countries featured. Because pre-hospital care is a rapidly developing profession and ambulance services are, in most places, constantly improving, I also acknowledge that some of my experiences would be quite different were I to have them now.

This book would not have been possible without funding from the Literature Board of the Australia Council for the Arts and a Sir Edward 'Weary' Dunlop Asialink Fellowship from the University of Melbourne. Generous material assistance was also provided by the professional association Australian College of Ambulance Professionals (ACAP) and Trek Medics International.

Sincere appreciation goes to Kevin Nutsford and my 'ambo' family at Bondi, to Jeff Gilchrist, Garren Constable, Giovanni Musillo, Dr Jason Bendall, Dr Rizwan Naseer, Dr Shiraz Afridi, Abdul Sattar and Bilquis Edhi, Hayat Khan, Vasif Shinwari, Farhan Arif, Birgir Finnsson, Andri Kjartansson, Erling Julinusson,

Sveinbjörn Berentsson, Señor X, Lars Svanstrom, Natasa Petkoska, Zoran Kostovski, Sinisa Davcevski, Dr Maja Poposka, Dr Lodovico Pietrosanti, Dr Manuela Silvestri, Mitzi Garcia Rodriguez, Dr Anton Padoan, Dr Michele Alzetta, Patty Dukes, Mark Rigg, Christopher 'Tippy' Lee, Mitch Kam, Jason Friesen and all the other ambulance medics who allowed me to share moments of their private and professional lives.

Thanks also goes to my agent James Wills and to publisher Scott Pack of The Friday Project for their enthusiasm and work on this international edition.

Finally, and most importantly, I wish to express my deepest gratitude to my beautiful and adventurous wife Kass and our precious daughter Paloma, the best travel companions a man could hope for; to the immensely supportive Warner family; and to my own wonderful parents, brothers and sister for their abundant love and encouragement.

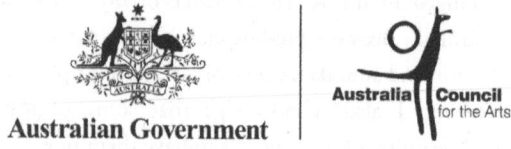

Australian Government

This project has been assisted by the Australian Government through the Australia Council, its arts funding and advisory body.

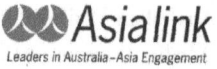

Leaders in Australia–Asia Engagement

For further information about Benjamin Gilmour and his projects, go to **www.paramedico.com.au** and www.benjamingilmour.com.

Milton Keynes UK
Ingram Content Group UK Ltd.
UKHW042037131024
449563UK00004B/139

9 780007 492510